OXFORD MEDICAL PUBLICATIONS

MEDICAL TRAVELLERS

MEDICAL TRAVELLERS

Narratives from the Seventeenth Eighteenth, and Nineteenth Centuries

———

JOHN D. SPILLANE
MD, FRCP

Oxford New York Toronto
OXFORD UNIVERSITY PRESS
1984

Oxford University Press, Walton Street, Oxford OX2 6DP

London Glasgow New York Toronto
Delhi Bombay Calcutta Madras Karachi
Kuala Lumpur Singapore Hong Kong Tokyo
Nairobi Dar es Salaam Cape Town
Melbourne Auckland
and associates in
Beirut Berlin Ibadan Mexico City Nicosia

Oxford is a trade mark of Oxford University Press

British Library Cataloguing in Publication Data
Spillane, John D.
Medical travellers.
1. Travellers   2. Physicians
I. Title
910'.92'2   G465
ISBN 0–19–261401–0

Library of Congress Cataloging in Publication Data
Spillane, John David.
Medical travellers.
(Oxford medical publications)
Bibliography: p.
Includes index.
1. Physicians—Great Britain—Biography. 2. Voyages
and travels. I. Title. II. Series.
R498.A1S64 1983   910.4   83–4260
ISBN 0–19–261401–0

Set by Promenade Graphics
Printed in Hong Kong

For
Jill, Sue, and Johnny

Preface

TRAVEL writing has been a field for all manner of men, doctors included. Keen scrutineers of the human face, trained, I was always told, in the art of 'sleuth-like observation', they might be expected to bring something distinctive to the genre. I cannot say that I have detected it, but there is certainly no question about their experience, down the ages, of leaving home. They have been at it for centuries. First, as itinerant students, later as practitioners or professors, often peddling a special message or cure, and nowadays zealous symposiasts commuting, not only to distant universities from Reykjavik to Rio and from Vancouver to Vellore, but also hurrying off to see a President or Maharajah, an oil-rich Sheikh or a loot-rich Dictator. Many a bar tale at a modern medical jamboree would have delighted Conrad, Kipling or Maugham—in whose hands it would have been fashioned into a story to be remembered.

But travellers' tales are only one aspect of travel writing. The subtitle of Oliver Goldsmith's poem *The Traveller*—the first publication issued in his own name and in which he was denoted 'M.B.'—was *A Prospect of Society*. His wanderings in Europe had left him with a tender appreciation of the spiritual and social relationships between the common man and his environment. In the journals on which this book is based one may catch a glimpse of this perspective. A few of these physician-travellers were celebrated, but apart from Smollett, their journals are unlikely to have been read by many modern readers. In briefly recalling them it is hoped that something of their flavour and spirit will give pleasure.

I wish to thank the following for helping me in my enquiries. Mr D. N. Cole, Librarian, Royal College of Physicians, London; Mr E. H. Cornelius, Librarian, Royal College of Surgeons, London; Mr D. W. C. Stewart, Librarian, Royal Society of Medicine, London; Mr N. H. Robinson, Librarian, The Royal Society, London; Joan S. Ferguson, Librarian, Royal College of Physicians, Edinburgh; Frances Sloan, Royal College of Physicians and Surgeons of Glasgow; Robert N. Smart, University Library, St. Andrews; Miss E. Talbot Rice, National Army Museum, London; Colonel A. V. Tennuci, RAMC Historical Museum, Aldershot; Mr M. J. Shepherd, National Maritime Museum, London; Sir Gordon Wolstenholme, Harveian Librarian, Royal College of Physicians, London; Professor J. A. Simpson, Department of Neurology, University of Glasgow; Dr. Robert M. Kark, Chicago; the staffs at the London Library; the National Library of Wales, Aberystwyth; the Baker Library and the Carpenter Library at Dartmouth College, New Hampshire, USA. For many of the photographic reproductions, I am indebted to Dr Ralph Marshall and his staff at the University Hospital of Wales, Cardiff, and to the photographic unit of the Royal Society of Medicine.

J. D. S.

Newport, Pembrokeshire
March, 1983

Acknowledgments

THE author and publishers are very grateful for permission to reproduce the following illustrations. Plate 1. Royal College of Physicians, London; Plate 4. *The Palaces of Leningrad*, by Victor and Audrey Kennett, Thames & Hudson, 1973; Plate 6. The Maryland Historical Society, Baltimore; Plates 8 and 9. The New York Public Library; Plate 10. The National Portrait Gallery, London; Plate 11. The Mansell Collection; Plate 12. The Pierpoint Morgan Library, New York; Plate 14. Royal Library, Windsor Castle, Reproduced by gracious permission of Her Majesty Queen Elizabeth II; Plate 17. Dorset Natural History and Archaeological Society, Dorset County Museum, Dorchester; Plate 19. The British Library, London; Plate 23. Royal Society of Medicine, London.

Contents

Contents

Plates

Plates

1

Introduction

BEFORE the seventeenth century few men, and still fewer women, voluntarily left home to travel abroad—except on pilgrimage or for reasons of health, business, or study, or in the service of the state. Travel, for pleasure was virtually unknown. The *reasons* for travel, Laurence Sterne waggishly observed in *A Sentimental Journey*, were ultimately derived from three general causes—'infirmity of the body, imbecility of mind, or inevitable necessity'. In the second class he seems to have included those who travelled 'labouring with pride . . . vanity or spleen'. His third class, 'the travellers of necessity'—the unwilling ones—comprised not only those 'delinquents travelling under the direction of governors recommended by the magistrate', but also those 'young gentlemen transported by the cruelty of parents and guardians and travelling under the direction of governors recommended by Oxford, Aberdeen or Glasgow'. These were in the custody of warders or tutors.

Travel usually required *permission* of one kind or another. In the days of Elizabeth I you could not leave England without the royal licence, and in the princedoms, kingdoms, and countries of Continental Europe, it was wise to carry letters of authorization or introduction, as well as a clutch of official warrants, permits, firmans or passports. Without them the traveller could land himself in all sorts of trouble. Not that they afforded any protection from hungry marauding peasants, robbers, disbanded mercenaries, bandits or, in the Mediterranean, African pirates. Nor from diseases like small-pox, dysentery, cholera, and rabies—not to mention the pox. Despite the hazards, the Grand Tour came to be regarded as an important, if not an indispensable, ingredient of a young gentleman's education.

As to its *value*, Francis Bacon had said that 'Travel, in the younger sort, is a part of education; in the older, a part of experience'. He advised the traveller to keep a diary and to 'sequester himself from the company of his countrymen'. Sterne said that 'An Englishman does not travel to see Englishmen'. In *The Art of Travel*, 1855, Francis Galton, that

Victorian polymath who abruptly relinquished his almost completed
medical studies and sailed for Africa, said that 'The scientific
advantages of travel are enormous . . . it is no slight advantage to a young
man, to have the opportunity for distinction which travel affords. If he
plans his journey among scenes and places likely to interest the
stay-at-home public, he will probably achieve a reputation that might
well be envied by wiser men who have not had his opportunities.' Dr
Henry Holland, as we shall see, was one such young man who realized
this and profited. How thrilled Galton would have been to read in our
British Medical Journal about the student electives roaming the globe.

The diaries and journals of travellers soon became popular reading;
publishers sought them and many were rescued from the libraries of
stately homes, colleges, vicarages and religious institutions. The
literature of travel blossomed in the eighteenth century and has
continued to be a favourite British avocation. In these days of mass
tourism, to travel vicariously with such splendid modern virtuousos as
Jan Morris and Patrick Leigh Fermor, is at times more rewarding,
certainly less wearying, than the real thing. When Tobias Smollett set
off, his luggage contained several trunks of books, among which were
four volumes of Nugent's *The Grand Tour*, published in 1743. As Italy
was the goal, the tour took on a classical aspect and many a don and
parson took up their pens. But Galton protested that 'owing to the
unhappy system of education that has hitherto prevailed, by which boys
acquire a very imperfect knowledge of the structure of two dead
languages, and none at all of the structure of the living world, most
persons preparing to travel are overwhelmed with the consciousness of
their incapacity to observe, with intelligence, the country they are about
to visit.'* Richard Bright was not one of these; he was artist and
geologist, as well as linguist.

Doctors had travelled, at first, in pursuit of education, mainly to such
universities as Montpellier, Padua, Leyden, and Paris. William Harvey
spent two years in Padua (1600–2) but left hardly any account of his
experiences. On the other hand, Felix Platter,† a medical student,
vividly recorded his adventures on his journeys from Basle to
Montpellier and back in the mid-sixteenth century. But generally
speaking, doctors have preferred writing autobiographies rather than
travelogues, although their travels, professional and otherwise, often
figure in their memoirs. But if one excludes the writings of explorers and

---

* Galton himself once used a sextant, trigonometry, and logarithms to measure a Hottentot
Venus at a safe distance (in his *Tropical South Africa*, 1853, p. 54).
   † *Beloved son Felix; the journal of Felix Platter* (trans. & ed. by Sean Jennett, 1961).

mountaineers, missionaries and colonial servants, and soldiers and sailors who were medical men, few doctors have contributed in an outstanding manner to the literature of travel—the exception being Tobias Smollett. Each of the following ten chapters is based on a book of travel written by a doctor. But I first wish to mention and comment on others which I have not selected for full consideration, for one reason or another, and which the reader may wish to consult. There are also doctors who travelled—like Oliver Goldsmith and Robert Graves—who regrettably left no adequate account of their experiences. They will be 'mentioned in dispatches'.

*

MARTIN LISTER (?1638–1712), a scholarly London physician, naturalist, and geologist, and one of Queen Anne's physicians, had found that his winter cough ceased when he went to France, so in 1698, he 'readily embraced' the opportunity of spending six months in Paris as a member of our embassy there. Although his book, published a year later, was entitled *A Journey to Paris*, he actually wrote only about the city itself, dealing in considerable detail with its lay-out, streets, squares, bridges, churches, convents, palaces, and gardens, and zealously listing the books, manuscripts, stamp collections, and 'curiosities, cabinets and rarities', he examined in the libraries, homes, and ecclesiastical houses he visited. The city was 'one of the most beautiful and magnificent in Europe'. more densely populated than London, with the people's dwellings crowded together because of the amount of ground taken up by palaces, convents, and gardens. It was 'a new city within this forty years' with houses built of stone—'walls, floors, staircases and all'—unlike London 'where every man that goes to bed, when asleep, lies like a dead Roman upon a funeral pile, dreading some unexpected apotheosis'. The streets were 'paved with a very great hard sand stone, each eight inches square', swept clean after snow 'by a heavy drag with a horse' and lit up at night 'all the winter long . . . by lanthorns in the very middle of the streets about twenty paces distance and twenty foot high'; they were made of iron and glass and each contained four large candles which burned till after midnight. Vandals who damaged them were 'forthwith sent to the galleys'.

The ease with which one could go by coach from the avenues into the fields and woods on every side was particularly delightful. 'The vast riding gardens are unknown to us in England . . . we cannot afford to lose so much country'. Some were 'twelve or fifteen miles in compass'. It seems that Louis XIV had by then developed an aversion to the Louvre and no longer relished Versailles and its air. Lister found him 'plump of face and well-coloured'; the king used to leave Versailles every Tuesday night for Marly, Meudon, or the Trianon, returning on Saturday night. The air of Paris was drier than that of England; registers had shown that 'there falls twice as much rain in England as at Paris'. He never saw a mist there and he noticed that iron did not rust in the miserable way it did in London. English grass was greener 'but we pay dearly for it, in agues and coughs, and rheumatic distempers'. In Paris there was such free 'insensible perspiration of the skin, that the kidneys had little to do'. You could drink wines freely 'yet they never broke your sleep to get shut of them'.

Only Parisians could drink the water from the local wells and the Seine without suffering from 'looseness and sometimes dysentery'. He did not believe that boiling it helped; visitors from other parts of France succumbed just as readily as did Lister's party, two-thirds of which 'fell into fluxes' within a month of their arrival. Bladder stone was very common and he saw many operations of 'cutting'; ten were completed in less than an hour by the monk *Frère* Jacques, the itinerant pioneer of this branch of surgery. Lister discovered that only sixteen out of forty-five survived his operation at the Hôtel Dieu and eleven out of nineteen at La Charité. Surgeons were critical and jealous of him 'though they practice his method'. But 'Pox here is the great business of the town'; quacks thrived, as in London, contributing to 'the ruin of physic'. All over Paris one could read advertisements for the cure of 'des malades secretes sans garder la chambre'. Everyone 'meddles with the cure of this disease, apothecaries, barbers, women and monks'. As in England, he said, physic was considered to be a 'knack, more than a science or method; and little chimical toys, the bijous of quacks, are mightily in request'.

There were dissections to watch, foetuses to examine, animals and plants to scrutinize, loadstones to experiment with, and *savants* of all kinds to consult. One topic that kept on cropping up was the circulation of the blood in the lungs. And there were reflections and anecdotes which reveal Lister as a kindly soul, with an unprejudiced outlook and possessing a pair of sharp eyes and ears. He was sorry that Monsieur S. 'rooked' the King at cards 'of near a million of livres', but sorry also that he had to be 'banished'. When describing the wan appearance of celibate monks in their strange habits, living 'on sour herbs, fish and such like trash', he thought it helped no one to renounce the world in this way; you simply renounced its blessings. He admired the lawyer 'who put himself at length into religion . . . but first persuaded his cook to do so too', and he wished that more monks had 'staid with their neighbours, and taught the world by their conversation and example'. He told 'the true story' of Molière dying suddenly 'in acting the *Malade Imaginaire* . . . saying, going off the stage, "Messieurs, J'ai joué *Le Malade Imaginaire*; mais je suis veritablement *fort Malade*"'. An old nobleman scholar who fell into a melancholy and died 'showed the first tokens of it by playing with a tame sparrow, and neglecting his mathematical schemes'. This led Lister to reflect that 'relaxation and unbending of the mind by innocent diversions' was a vital factor in preserving the health of the body and mind. Sleep, he thought, 'was nothing else that I know of, but the giving up the reins'.

We hear nothing of the vituperation later bestowed on the French by Smollett, but the English, Lister was told, were considered brave in war, civil in peace, 'curious and inquisitive after all good things . . . made a good judgement of what was commendable . . . and they [the French] did see a great difference between them and other nations'. He wrote up his journal, he said, 'to delight myself with the memory of what I had seen'.

*

OLIVER GOLDSMITH was forty-one and his friend Samuel Johnson sixty years of age, when they went to Oxford together on 14 February 1769, to receive honorary degrees. Goldsmith was granted the degree of Bachelor of Medicine and Johnson was honoured as a Doctor of Letters. Thirty-eight years had passed since Johnson had been forced by poverty to leave Pembroke College, after two years, without a degree. Goldsmith had studied for four years at Trinity College, Dublin, and had acquired the degree of Bachelor of Arts at the age of twenty. A few years later, in 1752, he took up the study of anatomy there, and then, in the autumn of that year, went on to Edinburgh. He enlisted in the anatomy class of Dr Monro, whom he thought the best teacher there and he attended lectures in chemistry, materia medica, and the theory and practice of physic. After sixteen months, anxious to continue his medical education abroad, he sailed, in February 1754, from Newcastle to Rotterdam, and went on to Leyden in a horse-drawn barge.

Delighted, at first, with the Dutch countryside and the comfortable mode of life of the people, he subsequently became bored and restless. There were only four British medical students there and teaching had declined since the days of the Boerhaave. As in Edinburgh, he was poor, not very diligent, and critical of the professors. He found the people too phlegmatic for his clownish taste. How long he actually spent in Leyden is not known—but it was probably about a year.

He took to the road and travelled on foot for nearly two years through Belgium, France, Germany, Switzerland, and Italy, visiting the university cities of Louvain, Paris, Geneva, Basle, and Padua, where he spent six months. Whether he supported himself, as he romantically claimed, by playing the flute in peasant homes in return for a meal, and by contributing to learned discussions of the classics and theology in various convents, or whether he was employed for some of the time as a travelling tutor, has never been confirmed. But he must have increased his knowledge of medicine, although there is no evidence that he acquired any medical degree—at Louvain or Padua—as he later implied and his early biographers wrote. Indeed , his submission to the University of Oxford, when he was admitted to their *ad eundem* degree in 1769, that he was already in possession of the Dublin degree of the Bachelor of Medicine, has never been substantiated.*

When he came to dictate material for a biography to his friend, the Reverend Thomas Percy, in 1773, the latter noted how Goldsmith's account of his years as a wandering student in Europe, resembled that of George Primrose, the son of his *Vicar of Wakefield*, published in 1766. This Percy memoir was incorporated into several editions of Goldsmith's *Collected Works*, beginning in 1801.

Destitute on his return to London in the summer of 1756, he hoped to be able to earn a living as a physician. At first he worked as assistant to apothecaries, but he failed to establish himself in practice in Southwark. Next came jobs as a schoolmaster and literary hack. In 1758 he failed to get a medical post with the East India Company or to pass the examination as a surgeon's mate at Surgeon's Hall. But by 1760 he was gaining more continuous employment as a journalist and essayist and there is evidence† that he was the author of an intelligent, unsigned review in *The Public Ledger* in 1761, of the Latin treatise *Inventum Novum*, published that year in Vienna by Auenbrugger. In it was described the technique and value of percussion of the chest in clinical medicine—a contribution which went unappreciated for fifty years.

Goldsmith's successful poem *The Traveller*, 1764, bore on its title page 'Oliver Goldsmith M.B.' and that year, at the suggestion of Sir Joshua Reynolds, he made a last attempt at medical practice—and

---

* See Sir Ernest Clarke, The medical education and qualifications of Oliver Goldsmith, *Proc. R. Soc. Med.*,7,88 (1914). Raymond Crawfurd, Oliver Goldsmith and Medicine, *Proc. R. Soc. Med.* 8, 7 (1915). John Ginger, *The Notable Man: the life and times of Oliver Goldsmith*. Hamish Hamilton London, (1977). J. B. Lyons, *The mystery of Oliver Goldsmith's medical degree*. Carraig Books, Blackrock, Co. Dublin (1978).

† See Saul Jarcho, A review of Auenbrugger's Inventum Novum, attributed to Oliver Goldsmith. *Bull. Hist. Med.* **33**, 470 (1969).

failed. Like Smollett, a decade or so earlier, he eventually found that his true métier was in the world of literature and not medicine.

But how enjoyable it would have been to read of the travels of a man who bequeathed to us of such masterpieces as *The Vicar of Wakefield*, *She Stoops to Conquer*, and *The Deserted Village*. That he did not write them is more of a loss to us than any academic shortcoming.

*

JOHN BELL (1763–1820), the Edinburgh surgeon, elder brother of Sir Charles Bell, spent the last three years of his life in Italy, dying in Rome of dropsy at the age of fifty-seven. In 1825 his wife published his *Observations on Italy*, a splendidly produced volume of 356 pages and dedicated to the King; it included twelve illustrations, two of them by the author (one is reproduced as Plate 13). The preface by his wife states that he had been ill and was seeking recovery of his health. In Paris, he wrote, 'I have seen much of the disappointments of life. I shall not feel them long'—his wife adding that there had been disappointments 'which tinged the colour of his whole life'.

These were references to his career in Edinburgh where he was educated and had practised. He was an anatomist and surgeon with a wide variety of talents at his disposal—an accomplished musician, a polished speaker, a popular lecturer, a skilled artist and a classical scholar. He was largely responsible for introducing surgical anatomy to the Edinburgh curriculum. He advocated dissection and not just demonstration, writing that 'In Dr Monro's class unless there be a fortunate succession of bloody murders, not three subjects are dissected in a year'. But his efforts to base surgery on anatomy and pathology were not welcomed; controversies arose and the professor of medicine finally ensured that only six surgeons were allowed to work at the Royal Infirmary—and Bell was not one of them. He actually taught for only thirteen years—from the ages of 23 to 36. But he became the leading surgeon in the city and remained so for thirty years, publishing several memorable volumes on anatomy, wounds, and the principles of surgery, all illustrated with drawings, etchings, and engravings by his own hand.

There is no portrait of him that I know, but he is said to have been of medium height, with a good figure and a pair of penetrating eyes; by nature he was energetic, 'impetuous', and in his disputations 'almost violent'. Some have thought that he should have left 'that windy and wordy city' and moved to London, as did so many Scottish doctors of his day, including his brother Charles. But the latter also became involved in bitter controversies about his researches. Neither of them had children.

There is little about Italy and the Italians in his book; most of it is about art and architecture, his wife expressing the hope that it might 'serve as a guide to the arts in Italy for young travellers'. He wrote with understanding in considerable detail about the paintings, frescoes, statues, palaces, museums, and churches in such cities as Turin, Milan, Florence, and Rome. His notes were made on the spot 'as he sat at the foot of a statue, on a stair, or on the height of a tower, from whence he contemplated the face of nature'.

In the refectory of the convent church in Milan he looked upon Leonardo da Vinci's 'Last Supper'—'a poor washy looking thing'— devoting seven pages to it and describing the attempts at restoration and the mistaken way the artist had originally prepared the ground layers on the wall on which it was painted. (He would have been delighted to learn how current restoration—the eleventh known one—is succeeding; the original painting is actually becoming visible.) There is an instructive account of the basic architecture of a typical Florentine palace; he concluded that the city's architects were 'masters of design, acquainted with geometry, optics, history, arithmetic and philosophy'. Some of his thoughts resemble those of Ruskin, later in the century, on the necessary equipment of the genuine art critic. Statuary, such as that of St. Bartholomew in Milan cathedral, the equestrian ones in the square in Piacenza, and the gladiators in Florence and Rome, were all examined closely from the anatomical as well as the artistic point of view; he was critical of some features. The statue of 'The Dying Gaul' in Rome filled him with 'feelings of admiration and sadness'; he visited it daily.

The scenic beauties of the landscapes, and the splendid sunsets in the cities or countryside, clearly moved him, but he said very little about the people. There are remarks about the clerics in the streets, wretched prisoners begging for bread through iron grills, and of crowds of peasants in a square or church ('There is nothing commendable in the Roman Catholic religion, but that the church is always open'). But the ladies of Modena were very attractive, possessing 'a natural elegance of figure . . . flexibility of limb and gracefulness of action', which made them popular as artists' models. He recorded nothing which amused him and we do not know where he stayed and how he fared; of Italian food and wine we learn nothing. There are no anecdotes or conversations or accounts of who he met, and but for the preface the reader would not know that he was accompanied by his wife.

Indeed, throughout the book there is a strain of melancholy. At the very start, on the road from Paris to Fontainebleau, he felt impelled to write that the beauty of a June morning helped 'in dispelling that undefined dejection of spirit, with which such powerful influence affects us at the outset of a long journey'. At Lyon we find that he had 'traversed all the meaner parts of Lyon, looked into their crooked alleys and staircases; examined what may be called hiding places for revolutionary hordes; and sought my way through dark courts, whose narrow staircases could emit hundreds of desperadoes . . . '. He dwelt on massacres which had been perpetrated there, and on a bridge disaster in which 238 people had perished—in 1711, over a century before. At Saint Foy there were the first of many 'gloomy subterranean vaults' and we hear of another massacre of Christians, this time, in the second century AD!

The word 'gloomy' recurs throughout his pages; there were gloomy church interiors, galleries and arcades and alcoves, roads and rivers, while even the 'architecture of Florence is grand and gloomy beyond that of all other cities in Italy'. The night he arrived in Turin he heard that there would be a public execution in the morning—'a beheading and breaking on the wheel'. The next morning we read that he 'found himself carried along in a crowd . . . to my suprise and horror I found myself exactly opposite the distracted criminal'. We read on for several pages about the condemned man in a black cart, half naked 'his countenance marked by strong and savage features . . . agonised with terror, every limb strained in anguish . . .' and the soldiers, priests, and chanting monks. Bell 'could not refrain from moralising upon the scene here presented', but to this reader his most interesting observation was that among the many thousands there, he counted only twenty females. Again, he chose to visit the Podesta prison in Florence, depicted in one of the engravings: there were 'engines of torture . . . bolts and bars of massive iron . . . grim pale faces worn by the ravages of disease . . . of those fit for the axe or guillotine'. He concluded by writing that he said to his conductors, 'I'll go no further . . . and left the place'.

The only hospital he mentioned was that at Lyon; 'it excelled everything I have ever seen'. There was a staff of 100 physicians and surgeons, and 150 nursing nuns, to care for 1000 patients. In Pavia medical school he met the famous Antonio Scarpa, like himself, artist and anatomist. They must have had an enjoyable meeting. He saw there some skulls of cretins—'the idiots of the Savoyard mountains'—and he noticed their large size and the thickness of the bone, and the manner in which they were all 'depressed at the great occipital pole, as if the head, being too heavy, had pressed to hard upon the *alba* . . . '. This must be one of the earliest observations of basilar invagination.

Of Italy as a whole, he wondered why, with its fine climate, its great rivers and seaports, and with such glorious art treasures, it had not achieved more power in the world, and why it had 'suffered itself to be the sport of contending and conflicting nations'. Perhaps, then, his last years were actually happier than a reader might have surmised.

According to Garrison (*History of Medicine*, 1917, 2nd edn, p.499) Bell's volume was 'one of the best books of travel written by a physician'. He also implied that Bell was responsible for the 'beautiful original drawings', some of which reminded him of Piranesi. It hardly amounts to that and, as I have said, only two of the illustrations were by Bell.

*

ROBERT JAMES GRAVES (1796–1853) was another Irish physician who, like Goldsmith, spent some years (1818–21) in Europe but left us no written record of his travels. This is particularly regrettable because he was a brilliant student who had had a classical as well as medical education at Trinity College, Dublin, and was an accomplished linguist, and writer on various topics of general interest as well as medical. His *Clinical Lectures on the Practice of Medicine*, 1843, was widely acclaimed throughout Europe and America, and he is remembered today in the term 'Graves' Disease' or toxic goitre.

We know that in his three postgraduate years he travelled in France, Germany, Switzerland, and Italy, visiting Paris, Berlin, Gottingen, Hamburg, Copenhagen, as well as cities in the north of Italy. If he had but kept a diary and subsequently taken up his pen and recounted his experiences, it would be surprising if, with his gifts, he would not have left us a valuable historical record of the Europe of his day. From time to time, in conversations, lectures, and essays, he mentioned certain of his observations—but written records are few.

Three anecdotes which give us a taste of what stories he might have told, are mentioned by William Stokes, his Dublin colleague, in his editorial introduction to a collection of Graves' essays—*Studies in Physiology and Medicine*, 1863. To illustrate Graves' 'remarkable power of acquiring languages' he said

On one occassion, when on a pedestrian journey in Austria, having neglected to carry his passport, he was arrested as a spy, and thrown into a dungeon. His assertion that he was a British subject was disbelieved by the authorities, who insisted that no Englishman could speak German as he did! In his imprisonment, which lasted for ten days, he suffered great privations.

Another episode was experienced on a brig in which Graves was sailing from Genoa to Sicily.

The captain and crew were Sicilians, and there were no passengers on board but himself and a poor Spaniard, who became his companion and messmate. Soon after quitting the land, they encountered a terrific gale from the north-east, with which the ill-found, ill-manned, and badly commanded vessel, soon showed herself unable to contend. The sails were blown away or torn, the vessel was leaking, the pumps choked, and the crew in despair gave up the attempt to work the ship. At this juncture Graves was lying on a couch in the cabin, suffering under a painful malady [this was a common way of referring to piles], when his fellow-passenger entered, and in terror announced to him that the crew were about to forsake the vessel; that they were then in the very act of getting out the boat, and that he had heard them say, that the two passengers were to be left to their fate. Springing from his couch, Graves flung on his cloak, and, looking through the cabin, found a heavy axe lying on the floor. This he seized, and concealing it under his cloak, he gained the deck, and found that the captain and crew had nearly succeeded in getting the boat free of its lashings. He addressed the captain, declaring his opinion that the boat could not live in such a sea, and that the attempt to launch it was madness. He was answered by an execration and told that it was a matter with which he had nothing to do, for that he and his companion should remain behind. 'Then', exclaimed he, 'if that be the case, let us all be drowned together. It is a pity to part good company'; as he spoke, he struck the sides of the boat with his axe, and destroyed it irreparably. The captain drew his dagger, and would have rushed upon him, but quailed before the cool, erect and armed man. Graves then virtually took command of the ship. He had the suckers of the pumps withdrawn, and furnished by cutting from his own boots, the leather necessary to repair the valves, the crew returned to their duties, the leak was gained, and the vessel saved.

Graves' meeting with J. M. W. Turner, the artist, is told as follows.

Graves was travelling by diligence, when, in one of the post-stations on the northern side of the Alps, a person took a seat beside him, whose appearance was that of a mate of a trading vessel. At first, no conversation took place between them, but Graves' curiosity was soon awakened by seeing his fellow-traveller take from his pocket a note-book, across the pages of which his hand, from time to time, passed with the rapidity of lightning. Overcome at length by curiosity, and under the impression that his companion was perhaps insane, Graves watched him more attentively, and discovered that his untiring hand had been faithfully noting down the forms of the clouds which crossed the sky as they drove along, and concluded that the stranger was no common man. Shortly afterwards, the travellers entered into conversation, and the aquaintance thus formed soon became more intimate. They journeyed together, remaining for some time in Florence, and then proceeding to Rome. Graves was himself possessed of no mean artistic powers and his sketches from nature are full of vigour and truth. He was one of the few men in whose company Turner is known to have worked. The writer has heard him describe how, having fixed on a point of view, he and his companion sat down, side by side to their work. 'I used to work away', he said 'for an hour or more, and put down as well as I could every object in the scene before me, copying form and colour, perhaps as faithfully as was possible in the time. When our work was done, and we compared drawings, the difference was strange; I assure you there was not a single stroke in Turner's drawing that I could see like nature; not a line nor an object, and yet my work was worthless in comparison with his. The whole glory of the scene was there'. The tone and fire with which Graves uttered these last few words, spoke volumes for his sympathy with and his admiration of the great painter of nature.

At times, however, when they had fixed upon a point of view, to which they had returned day after day, Turner would often content himself with making one careful outline of the scene. And then, while Graves worked on, Turner would remain apparently doing nothing, till at some particular moment, perhaps on the third day, he would exclaim 'There it is!' and seizing his colours, work rapidly until he had noted down the peculiar effect he wished to fix in his memory. It is a curious fact, that these two remarkable men lived and travelled together for months, without either of them inquiring the name of his comrade, and it was not till they reached Rome, that Graves learned that his companion was the great artist.

Turner was forty-four when, in 1819, he visited Italy for the first time. He left no autobiography or memoir of his tours abroad and the majority of his letters are not very interesting. But in the recently published *Collected Correspondence of J. M. W. Turner* (Clarendon Press, Oxford 1980, edited by John Gage), in which there are many of his hitherto unpublished letters, I was, for a moment, delighted to see the name of Robert Graves in the index. Alas, it did not refer to the physician, but to an engraver of London. One would have enjoyed discovering the artist's account of his meeting with Graves the physician.

*

MARSHALL HALL (1790–1857) was another famous doctor whose wife published an account of their travels; *Memoirs of Marshall Hall*, 1861. He graduated in Edinburgh in 1812 and studied for some time on the continent before settling in practice in Nottingham. He went on to Gottingen and Berlin from Paris, his wife recording that he did the journey alone, on foot, a distance of 600 miles, in the month of November 1814. He moved to London in 1826 where he developed an extensive practice in Mayfair. Although he lectured from time to time at various hospitals and institutions, he was never appointed to the staff of a London hospital. He was an indefatigable researcher and prolific writer, establishing that the reflex was an essential feature of all nervous activity. He was elected FRS in 1832. He had many a quarrel with other scientists and doctors, some arising from his exaggerated claims, others from lack of acknowledgement of the work of others, and actual plagiarism. He indulged in endless vituperative tirades, paranoid in tone, and his wife referred to the 'persecution', 'jealousies', 'prejudices', and 'injustices' he had experienced, and how 'no honours were ever conferred on him in England', but how widely he was acclaimed in Europe and America.

To the general reader his name may recall his technique of artificial respiration in cases of drowning which was adopted by the National Lifeboat Institution. It may also bring to mind that other Marshall Hall (1858–1927), Sir Edward, the eminent barrister. Sir Edward was not his son contrary to what has often been said; they were not related. Dr Marshall Hall was attended in his last illness by a Dr Alfred Hall, in Brighton, who asked permission to name a son after the famous neurologist. The son, born shortly after the doctor's death, became the barrister.

Throughout his twenty-six years of London practice, Hall and his wife travelled each year in Europe—'at the end of the London season'—as did Sir Henry Holland, who, as we shall see, also practised in Mayfair without a hospital appointment. The widow's *Memoir*, of some 500 pages, is essentially a long eulogium about her husband's near-saintly character, his researches, and his good works (he campaigned against bloodletting, flogging in the army, and for better schemes for sewage disposal). Their yearly trips abroad were of a conventional nature and are described in sentimental Victorian prose which a modern reader would not find of much interest. But she devoted a long chapter to an account of a fifteen-month tour which they made with their son in North America, Canada and Cuba in 1853–4, on his retirement from practice at the age of sixty-three. It is not without interest, although larded with references to the fame which had preceded him, the rapturous applause accorded his lectures and the hospitality they enjoyed.

He had read De Tocqueville's *De la Démocratie en Amérique* (1835) and throughout the tour the question of slavery was repeatedly discussed. Characteristically, during the eleven-day crossing by steamship from Liverpool to New York, he found time to write a paper on seasickness, which was promptly published in the *Comptes Rendus* of the Institute of France. In Washington he was impressed 'by the simple pageantry of the inauguration of Mr Franklin Pierce as President of the United States' and in Baltimore he was so fêted that his proposed stay of five days was extended to twenty-one. After two weeks in Philadelphia they felt in America 'a spirit of unanimity seems to pervade the *corps médical*'; 'disparaging remarks' were never heard. They went by railroad across the Appalachians to Pittsburgh and then down the Ohio river for 500 miles to Cincinnati. From there, another day's steaming down the Ohio brought them to Louisville, Kentucky. Taking a respite from his lecture-demonstrations, for which he was amply supplied with frogs and snakes (and later in the tour, with an alligator), the Hall family rode for three days in a carriage to visit the Mammoth Caves, in the centre of the State. Now a well-known tourist attraction, they consisted of an extensive system of limestone caves which covered an area of 150 square miles. The Hall son penetrated a distance of ten miles, presumably with a guide, and Mrs Hall put on her 'bloomer costume', as she had done on similar explorations of European caves.

During their weeks in Kentucky, Hall developed his ideas for a gradual emancipation of slaves and a paper on his scheme was published in the *Louisville Journal*, with an understanding comment by its editor.

Continuing their journey down the Ohio they came to its junction with the Mississippi, at what is now the city of Cairo, and turned up that river to reach St. Louis, Missouri, in three days. After further lectures and visits, they went up river for several hundred miles to 'the new small town' of St. Paul, Minnesota, where railway engineering prospectors were setting out to explore a route through the Rocky mountains to California. They were told that west of St. Paul there was no real town till one reached California. They visited among the Sioux and Winnebago Indians and with the Governor of the territory and a military escort they went up river for 80 miles to a conference with the Chippewas and others. There had been some 'difficulties and scalping affairs'.

Turning south down the Mississippi again as far as Galena, just south of Dubuque, they took a carriage across the prairie to Chicago, a distance of 160 miles. The railroad had not been built yet and sections of the road were called 'corduroy' because they were made of logs laid side by side across the road—as travellers in Russia had described. A voyage, across the Great Lakes to Buffalo, took five days.

Niagara, Hall thought, came fourth in his list of the most beautiful natural scenes he had seen; after Mont Blanc, the glacier of Argentière and Vesuvius. At a lecture in Buffalo, an ex-President of the United States—a Mr Millard Fillmore—was in the audience (I suppose that most readers, like myself, have never heard of the two Presidents mentioned).

The Canadian cities of Hamilton, Montreal, Toronto, and Quebec were next visited, and then they turned southwards once again and passed via Lake Champlain, Saratoga, and Albany to the Hudson river, West Point, and New York. Lectures there and in Boston were to follow, before they began a second circuit through the South—Virginia, the Carolinas, Alabama, Georgia, and Louisiana. From New Orleans, where Hall witnessed a slave being severely flogged, they sailed to Havana, Cuba. There, he lectured in French and found the students eager and gentlemanly. They were not able to sail on to New York because of a customs dispute between Spain and the United States, and were forced to return to New Orleans. From there to New York took twenty days, eight of them steaming up the Mississippi and Ohio rivers to Louisville. From there they continued on the Ohio to Cincinnati, and then by railroad to Buffalo and New York.

Dr Hall wrote many letters home about slavery, and on his return he published a small book entitled '*The twofold slavery of the United States*', in which he proposed a scheme of gradual 'self-emancipation with due preparation by education'.

Not an exciting travelogue perhaps, but an early example of medical travel in the New World—a development which, in due course, grew and flourished, acquiring in the medical world something of the prestige of *The Grand Tour* itself.

*

OLIVER WENDELL HOLMES (1809–94), in his seventy-seventh year, decided that after an interval of fifty years, he would take 'a second look at Europe'. He had known it as a medical student in Paris in the years 1833–35, when the voyage from New York to Portsmouth had taken twenty-four days. He rode on the only railroad he saw in Europe—Manchester to Liverpool. 'I looked upon England from the box of a stage-coach, upon France from the coupé of a diligence, upon Italy from the cushion of a carozza.' On his return to Boston, he graduated in medicine, began practice in the city, and was soon also appointed as a professor of anatomy and physiology at Dartmouth College. From 1847 to 1882 he held a similar post in Harvard Medical School. He once said that his various duties made him think that he occupied 'not a chair but a settee'. In 1843, five years before Semmelweis, he established that puerperal fever was contagious, a discovery for which, after a period of abuse, he was subsequently honoured. When ether was first used in surgery in Boston, in 1846, he coined the word 'anaesthesia'.

Witty and sociable, a splendid conversationalist, he had 'first tasted the intoxicating pleasure of authorship' as a student, contributing to a college journal. 'There is no form of lead-poisoning which more rapidly and thoroughly pervades the blood and bones and marrow than that which reaches the young author through mental contact with typemetal.' He became a literary figure in 1857 on the appearance of the first papers of the *Autocrat of the Breakfast Table* in *The Atlantic Monthly*, a magazine of which he was one of the founders and which he actually christened. Later, there were the *Professor*; the *Poet*; and novels, verses, and essays.

Our Hundred Days in Europe, the title of the book he wrote about his return visit in 1886, describes what must have been a particularly delightful academic-aristocratic joy-ride through England—a Victorian Cavalcade. He received honorary doctorates at Oxford, Cambridge and Edinburgh, he was entertained at Windsor, Westminster, at the Foreign Office, at Royal Garden Parties, at numerous stately homes, and at Epsom. He enjoyed a perpetual round of social engagements— breakfasts, lunches, teas, and dinners. Titled ladies galore flit or saunter across his pages. At Compton Wynyate he recited a few poems to an audience which included a Marquis and his Lady; he stayed with Lord Tennyson at Farringdon, in the Isle of Wight. He found relaxation and interests at Chester, York and Stratford, at Salisbury, Stonehenge, Old Sarum and Brighton, and at Malvern, and Tewkesbury, and Bath. Everything was splendid everywhere—except the weather. He was 'entirely disenchanted with it'—May and June were cold and wet.

In Paris, there is a wistful, even a sombre note at times. August was 'the dead season'; the solitude of familiar places like the Place Vendôme he found oppressive—not actually 'melancholic', like 'Oliver Goldsmith by the lazy Scheld or wandering Po' in *The Traveller*. He did not venture into the Hôpital Pitié—he had not practiced medicine for forty years—but remembered his revered teacher there, Pierre Louis, who was 'idolised' by American students. In the Paris of his student days, a stethoscope was 'almost a novelty' and he never saw a microscope. He called on Pasteur, sending in a card on which he had written that he was an American physician 'who wished to look in his face and take his hand'.

His *Hundred Days* may not amount to much in the actual field we are scanning, and he did not think it was exactly 'A Sentimental Journey', but it was written with humour, imagination, and tenderness, entirely free of that era's pomposity. Its tone, in fact, recalls the Autocrat's engaging opening line of thirty years before—'I was just going to say, when I was interrupted, that one of the many ways of classifying minds is under the heads of arithmetical and algebraical intellects'.

*

SIR FREDERICK TREVES (1853–1923) was the London surgeon who reputedly told King Edward VII, reluctant to postpone his coronation, that if he did not allow him to remove his inflamed appendix, 'Then, Sir, you will go as a corpse'. But he is remembered today as the author of *The Elephant Man*, a tale that took up only twenty pages in a short volume of reminiscences published in 1923, the year he died. But for some twenty years he had been writing about his travels, beginning with a round-the-world trip, and followed by books on Dorset, the Caribbean, Uganda, the Holy Land, Italy, the Riviera, and Lake Geneva. He wrote with fluency, in a down-to-earth manner and had a keen eye for scene and character.

The first of these books, in 1905, was entitled *The other side of the lantern; an account of a commonplace tour round the world*, a volume of some 420 gilt-edged pages, illustrated with forty of his photographs (a surprising number of which are unpeopled and have a deserted look, as in those of his book on the Riviera), splendidly bound in embossed leather and dedicated to King Edward. His preface ran

A paper lantern, round and red, hangs under a cloud of cherry blossom in a Japanese village. There is a very familiar flower symbol painted upon one side of it. Some children have crossed the green to see what is on the other side of the lantern. A like curiosity has led to the writing of this trivial book.

A bit 'high-falutin' to modern eyes, but sentiment pervades his pages. He went by sea to India and then travelled on to Burma, Ceylon, Singapore and Penang, Hong Kong, Canton, Shanghai, Japan, Honolulu, and America. He obviously wished his book to be more than a trite record of his tour. His chapter headings are an indication—Port Said was *The Stage Villain's Town*—Benares was *The City of Trampled Flowers*—Burmese women were *The Ladies of Creation*—a Kyoto temple was *The St. Peter's of Japan*. His final chapter—*The Scene of the End of the World*—was about the Grand Canyon. He seems to have felt that 'the rent is fresh, that the world has burst asunder but yesterday . . . here is the scene of a terrific world-ending catastrophe'. But geologists tell us that the river Colorado has been the principal agent; the river cutting vertically downwards and the plateau gradually rising.

This decorative style is accompanied by a liberal sprinkling of poetic quotations and old saws such as—'Those who go down to the sea in ships' (page 1)—'They toil not neither do they spin'—'There is a green hill far away'—Faithful unto death'—'The peace that passeth all understanding'—'Sermons in stone, and good in everything' and 'The great world spins forever down the ringing grooves of change'. On his final page when the inevitable 'white cliffs' are glimpsed again—with 'kindly-tended fields . . . sturdy English oaks . . . and ivied towers'—he finishes with a verse from Kipling's *Sussex* about God giving 'all men all earth to love'.

But all this, although dating the book, goes with some good pieces of observation and well-captured scenes. As at Heathrow today, the crowds and confusion at Tilbury were a regrettable aspect of 'modern change'. But he was able to spot, or imagine, the 'widow' who had come to see her 'only' son off to India, crouching on the pierside as the ship moved off, while her son was already in the bar telling how much money 'he has screwed out of the old mater'. At Port Said, where the boys called every man 'Mr. Gladstone' and every lady 'Mrs. Langtry', the touts sold 'postcards' and importuned men to visit 'a dancing saloon'. Coaling the ship there is vividly described. It went on through the night, lit up by flares, with port holes closed, rough canvas covering stairs and corridors, and with everyone trying to escape the noise and coal dust. The coal was carried by arabs and negroes in yellow baskets from huge barges alongside—up one plank and down another in an endless stream. In India 'An elephant moving appears to be extraordinarily full of joints; his tread is spongy like an old butler'. A Burmese girl emerging from a wood was 'a brilliant little personage, graceful in her slightest movement, infinitely feminine, full to her lips with the sparkle of life, yet dignified and even stately'.

Hong Kong looked as if it were 'made up of Hull, Monte Carlo, and a Derbyshire hill' where you had 'to learn how to breath steam . . . to see the world through the atmosphere of a laundry, to write on damp paper, to keep your gloves in bottles and to sit still and drip', presumably in London clothes and stiff collars. Kyoto was 'a wide city of pewter-grey roofs, jumbled together about the same dull level, as if it were a pond grown over with stiff grey leaves which had been tilted by the wind at many angles'. In a Japanese temple he saw a girl tying a little knot of paper, carrying a prayer for a husband, to a grating, using only the thumb and little finger of one hand. This explained an observation he had made in a tea-house—a girl, alone, endlessly practising this tricky manoeuvre.

The Chinese, though 'terrified of foreigners', were 'men of the world'. In any climate, they could tackle any job. The Japanese 'appear to be easy-going and unbusinesslike, while those who have lived long with them speak of their hosts as 'casual and sketchy' and 'incapable of great intellectual effort'. Yet Treves observed how skilfully they were conducting their war in Russia, which had broken out while he was in Penang. He knew they were acutely imitative 'but they have improved whatever they have copied'. He could not understand why the most artistic people in the world were content to export so much shoddy goods. Japanese soldiers impressed him; entraining for the front, there was none of the shouting and drunkenness, 'no swagger of bravado', so familiar at home; a victory parade carried 'none of the savage cult of "mafficking"' The army medical services were efficiently organized; prevention of illness was the goal. Treves had served in the Boer war and he wrote that 'It is a little distressing to reflect how many lives might have been saved if the methods of the Japanese Medical Service had been adopted by the British Army'. He anticipated a great future for Japanese surgery.

More than a third of the volume is devoted to India, the governing of which was 'a wonderous thing to contemplate . . . but at what a cost in British lives'. Cantonment life, with its yearning for home is described and the main epics of the Indian Mutiny retold—the massacre at Cawnpore, the siege of Lucknow, the Kashmir Gate, and the Delhi Ridge, but at the end, no thought whether there would ever be an end to British rule. Perhaps it would not have been seemly for the Sergeant-Surgeon to H.M. the King to dwell on such a matter. Far better to mention, in passing, how well each governor was doing and how popular was his lady. (In Burma she 'maintained a popularity as hearty as her husband's'; in Hong Kong she was 'the most popular lady in the island'.) In Simla, they had built 'a little piece of Britain', just as, today, the American, in his overseas hotels and 'cantonments', recreates his home environment, with Coca Cola and peanut butter taking the place of tea and marmalade.

And so, Sir Frederick proceeded round the world, noting 'the wind of change' (his words), always observant and sometimes sentimental, but never with the slightest hint of self-esteem. As an Edwardian there were things he would not mention, such as the nature of the postcards and dancing saloons at Port Said, or the breasts of the girls in Burma or Ceylon. Eyes, waists, limbs—yes, but no more. Sea bathing, too, was still 'a rudimentary pursuit', even in Honolulu. And as for the female role in this world—'the blue-stocking lecturer on women's rights . . . with a creaking voice and a bony and mittened fist'—is contrasted unfavourably with the native lady's 'amiable capacity and a readiness to undertake loyally whatever the particular hand may find to do'. Which last, may explain why the reader does not learn, until towards the end of the book, that Sir Frederick was accompanied on his journey, by his wife and daughter. Their sole appearance is when, in Tokyo, they had an audience with the Empress of Japan. Sir Frederick had one with the Emperor as well. I have not read all his travel books, but they were popular and well received. Three of them remain quite enjoyable—*The Land that is desolate* (The Holy Land)—*The Riviera of the Corniche Road*—and *The Lake of Geneva.*

*

Lastly before introducing our ten authors, there is one other—*Sir George Lefevre* (1798–1846)—who may be mentioned in passing—but not in despatches. The very title of his three volume work—*The Life of a Travelling Physician; from his first introduction to practice; including twenty years wandering through the greater part of Europe* (1843)—suggests he would surely be among the chosen few. But Lefevre admitted that his book was 'a curious production, touching upon many things and dwelling upon none' and he said that a friend who was asked for a candid opinion of the manuscript, replied—'My candid opinion, Sir? . . . I consider it one of those works which gives the author much more pleasure in the composition than any profit he can hope for by the sale of it'. And with similar thoughts I think we can leave him for others to pursue—and pick up the trail of our quarry.

*

Our ten chosen medical travellers were all British, two of them illustrious physicians whose names—RICHARD BRIGHT (1789–1858) and THOMAS HODGKIN (1798–1866)—are remembered eponymously in the terms 'Bright's disease' and 'Hodgkin's disease'; Bright's journey was in Hungary in 1815 and Hodgkin's in Morocco in 1863. The third TOBIAS SMOLLETT (1721–71), was never a very successful practitioner of medicine, but, with Richardson and Fielding, he was one of the creators of the English novel, in the eighteenth century; his travel journal about France and Italy is a gem. DR EDWARD BROWNE (1644–1708), son of Sir Thomas Browne the celebrated author of *Religio Medici*, was physician to Charles II and a President of the Royal College of Physicians. He travelled extensively in Europe in 1668–9. Our fifth author SIR HENRY HOLLAND (1788–1873) was also and eminent person, physician to Queen Victoria and a President of the Royal Institution; his book was about Greece and Albania in 1812–13.

The five remaining men would not be remembered but for their five books. JOHN BELL of Antermony (1691–1780) made several long journeys in Russia and Central Asia, and one as far as Peking, between 1715 and 1737. ALEXANDER HAMILTON (1712–56) went on horseback from Maryland to Maine in 1744. JOHN WHITE was a surgeon in the Royal Navy who sailed in the first fleet which transported convicts to Botany Bay in 1787; he was made Surgeon-General to the first settlement there. WILLIAM WITTMAN was surgeon to the British military mission to Constantinople in 1799 and he went with the Turkish army across Palestine to Egypt during Bonaparte's campaign there. CLARKE ABEL (1780–1826) was surgeon to the second British Embassy to Peking in 1816.

For Browne and Bright, their journeys were primarily educational, while Hamilton and Smollett were seeking relief from chest complaints, probably tuberculous. Hodgkin travelled as a physician and friend to a wealthy philanthropist. Bell and Holland were born travellers for whom new faces and places were the breath of life. Six of them—Browne, Bell, Hamilton, Holland, Bright, and Abel—were in their twenties; White and Wittman probably in their thirties; Smollett was forty-two, and Hodgkin sixty-five. They all died in their beds, though not necessarily at home. Smollett died in Leghorn, Wittman in Paris, Abel in Calcutta, and Hodgkin in Jaffa. Two of them lived to a great age—Bell to eighty-nine and Holland to eighty-five.

Aside from the general scenes they described, several of them were witnesses of historical developments and events. Bell saw the building of St. Petersburg by Peter the great; White the founding of the first colony in Australia; Wittman the surrender of the French in Egypt. Bright was a spectator of that Machiavellian symposium—the Congress of Vienna. Or take the state of the countries they visited. Browne crossed Germany twenty years after the devastation of the Thirty Years War and commented on the striking degree of recovery which had taken place so that 'the effects were scarcerly discernable'. And in France, twenty-five years before the revolution, Smollett foretold the inevitable dangers of punitive taxation, an oppressed peasantry, an aristocracy ignorant of agriculture, and he sensed that 'a spirit of freedom takes the ascendant'. From Hamilton, in the American colonies three decades before the War of Independence, we glimpse a picture of the social life which is quite unique.

Four of our five nineteenth century travellers provided maps of their
routes—Wittman, Holland, Bright and Abel. Bell was the only earlier
traveller to do so, but his map (p. 54) showing how he went from
Moscow to Peking, though picturesque and interesting, is understand-
ably a crude presentation. In drawing new maps, I have traced as
accurately as I could, all the journeys which were undertaken. No
practised cartographer, this was none the less enjoyable, although some
of the tasks were a trifle laborious so that I wished for a young lady at my
side—with a keener eye and a steadier hand. Bell's spelling of place
names, he confessed, was largely phonetical—*Shamachy* for Shemakha,
for example. With Bell, too, there was the perplexing problem of
changes in place names over the years; Kuybyshev for *Samara*, Gorky or
Gorkiy for *Nishna-Novogorod*, Molotov for *Solikamsky*, and Stalingrad
for *Czaritza*. In central Europe and the Balkans, the names used by
Browne have been replaced by ones which recognize the ethnic origin of
the peoples. And in Greece, the spelling of the place names continues to
vary. Particularly striking are the changes which have occurred in
Bright's map of Hungary; Bratislava (now in Czechoslovakia) for
Pressburg, Vac for *Waitzen*, Gyor for *Raab*, Pecs for *Funfkirchen*, and so
on. I have drawn modern national boundaries and used names and
spelling which seemed most familiar.

In the British Isles, place names have thankfully remained much the
same for centuries, and except for bureaucratic innovations and gusts of
national pride, we have not had to endure Central Europe's recurring
rechristening of cities, towns, villages, rivers, mountains. In reading
these narratives and drawing my maps one has come to appreciate more
clearly how geography influenced the siting of towns and the routes
taken by men, with goods or weapons, as they moved or migrated across
the land. The touring motorist of today is likely to use a map which is
nothing more than a network of lines of many colours in which the
course of a river may be effectively concealed. Old maps are better.
Before the automobile there was space on them to display the contour of
the land so that one could see how men came to use certain highways
and waterways in peace and war.

Overland travellers, on foot or on horseback, could of course take to
the rivers for part of their journey. There were ferries galore for
Hamilton to cross on his way up to New York. Highways between the
Rhine and the Danube were of ancient importance; Browne went via
Nuremberg to reach the Danube at Regensburg, and recalled Charlemagne's attempt to build a canal between the two rivers, which would
have provided a waterway from the North to the Black Sea, a project still

being pursued.* In Russia Bell found that in winter a horse-drawn sleigh could cover 500 miles in three days. On the way to Isfahan he went down the Volga for a thousand miles. In the mountains of Greece and Albania, Holland, a good horseman, had many an arduous ride. He said that a Tartar horseman could ride from Yanina in Albania, to Constantinople in six days—about 500 miles as the crow flies. Browne used only one horse in his solitary ride of 350 miles from Venice to Vienna. Coaches—with four wheels, springs, and a roof—came into use in the sixteenth century; Smollett bowled along in diligence or berline on some good French roads, and Bright illustrated the crude type of wagon in which he was conveyed on the muddy tracks of the Hungarian plains.

We also catch a glimpse of some of the old-established overland trade routes in these narratives. There were the long classical caravan routes from India across Central Asia to the Caspian and the Mediterranean; in Isfahan Bell met a Dutch Governor returning from Batavia and on the Volga he saw the gigantic barges used for transporting salt which required a crew of six to eight hundred oarsmen and towmen. In China, Abel voyaged from Peking to Canton about 1400 miles, almost entirely by water; first via the Grand Canal between the Pei-ho and the Yangtse, down that river, and into the Kan. As on the Volga, the Yangtse barges were towed by men who sang songs of sadness and hunger. In Salonika, Holland saw great horse-caravans setting out for Vienna, via Bulgaria and Budapest, a journey which took thirty-five days.

And the people? Well they interested some travellers more than others. Hodgkin had little to say but Smollett never ceased to upbraid them—French arrogance and Italian untrustworthiness being fully recorded in vituperative fashion. Browne found the Dutch industrious and marvelled at what they had accomplished, Wittman would have been happy to live among them, but Hamilton, in Albany, found them unattractive—the women dowdy and the men concerned only with 'profits'. Bright and Browne recognized the superior industry and reliability of the Germans. Hungarian landowners, said Bright, were excellent agriculturalists but treated their peasants as slaves; Slovakians were wretched looking. In Moravia, Browne found the people 'plain dealing, stout and making good soldiers' and in Bohemia they were intelligent and active, good horsemen, skilled at mining. In Saxony the common folk were rough and boisterous; they drank too much but were

* Negley Farson in *Sailing across Europe* (1930), went down the Rhine and used the old forgotten Ludwig Canal from the Main up over the Juras to Nuremberg, and thence down the Altmuhl to the Danube.

civil to strangers. But it was the Tartars whom Bell found the most attractive—gay, hardy, honest, and reliable. He speaks of them with affection, as we still do of the Gurkhas. Chinese peasants, Abel found, were helpful and pleasant but the merchants were greedy.

Jews were also referred to in many places—Amsterdam, Frankfurt, Vienna, Salonika, and Russia. Their ghettos were outside or inside the city walls, and they had to obey curfews and wear distinctive hats or dress. They were best treated in Holland, where they thrived; they were expelled from Vienna shortly after Browne's visit. Many of the itinerant traders seen on the roads of Central Europe were Jewish. And it was the plight of Jews in Morocco that took Hodgkin there. In general, Turks were the most fearsome warriors and Arabs the most inveterate thieves. Gypsies, thought Bright, resembled the Jews in the way in which they had preserved their language and customs while wandering for centuries over the lands of Europe. Fierce dogs plagued Bell, Wittman, and Holland.

Aside from the occasional British travellers our doctors met on the roads, there were the expatriated who turned up in the most unlikely of places. There was the English engineer in Stalingrad, building a canal between the Don and the Volga; the carpenter with a Tartar wife in Kazan; a Scottish apothecary in Ljubljana; a merchant in Salonika who had been there for thirty years; and in Cairo a 'General of Bombardiers' who had served with the Turkish forces for fifty years—a Scot, of course name of Campbell.

The pages of Hamilton's journal are alive with characters of all kinds—landlords, servants, maids, ferrymen, parsons, dons, quacks, tinkers, old soldiers, and rogues—all full of talk and nonsense of endless variety. One old fellow in Newport, Rhode Island, explained how a canal could be cut through the isthmus at Panama and ships drawn through from the Atlantic to the Pacific! Hamilton's journal is as readable, as Smollett's but not, of course, as wide-ranging in history, and as scholarly,—and his humour is always cheerful and good-natured.

But in them all, in addition to the general panoramas depicted, one comes across items of observation which surprise or intrigue. There is Browne's description of the chairs which revolved round a dining table in Dortrecht, so that the diners could gain a good view of the surroundings. Then there was Bell noting the bituminous oil near Baku, and Hodgkin, the plateau of phosphates in Morocco. Smollett's description of the collecting of human manure in Nice, and the comparison between the products of Catholic and Protestant households, is hilarious. But Abel takes it further with his description of how the Chinese deodorized, packaged, and dispatched the stuff all over China. The story of the convict coiners at Rio made one wish they had succeeded—as did so very few escapees in Botany Bay. The continuing popularity of Gensing comes to mind when mentioned by Hamilton and Abel.

At the end there linger a few thoughts about items not mentioned—such as windmills in Holland and Leeuwenhoek in Delft, by Browne; the witches of Salem by Hamilton; Peter the Great's epilepsy by Bell; acupuncture by Abel. And in Richard Bright's Vienna why do we hear nothing of Bach, Handel, Haydn, Mozart, Schubert—and only a passing reference to a minor piece of music by Beethoven? One book leads to another. Interests vary, but some readers of these journals (or even perhaps of my book) may be tempted to look further into these times and events of which they speak. For myself, I found Browne leading me to The Thirty Years War; Bell, to Peter the Great; White, to early Australia; Wittman, to the French in Egypt; and Holland, to the Greek struggle for independence.

2

Dr Edward Browne's Travels in Europe in the Seventeenth Century 1668–1669

EDWARD BROWNE (1644–1708) was the eldest son of Sir Thomas Browne, a physician of Norwich and author of *Religio Medici*—the religion of a physician. This was written shortly after he had returned from Europe where he had been studying medicine at Montpellier, Padua, and Leyden, where he had obtained the degree of doctor of medicine. The book reflected the impressions made on his mind by the bigotry he had met with in catholic Italy and protestant Holland. It achieved widespread celebrity for its literary style and liberality of sentiment, notwithstanding some criticism by Dr Johnson. He thought that although it was learned, it was pedantic and obscure, 'a tissue of many languages, a mixture of heterogeneous words brought together from distant regions'.

Edward Browne went to school in Norwich and entered Trinity College, Cambridge when he was thirteen, graduating bachelor of medicine six years later. After some months with his father in Norwich, studying and dissecting, he went to London and attended some lectures at St. Bartholomew's Hospital. In 1664 he travelled in France and Italy with a few distinguished young Englishmen, one of whom was Christopher Wren. His account of this journey was never published, except for a portion of it which was included in the folio edition of his travels. The original manuscript is preserved in the Sloane MSS in the British Museum.

On his return to England he studied medicine at Oxford, proceeding to doctor of medicine in 1667, and also being admitted a Fellow of the recently created Royal Society of London. He was twenty-four years of age when he began the travels for which he was remembered. He left England in August 1668 and travelled to Vienna. From there, in 1669, he made three journeys—to Hungary, Venice, and Greece. He travelled homewards across Germany, reaching London at the end of December, 1669.

He then settled in London, became a Fellow of the Royal College of Physicians and was elected to the staff of St. Bartholomew's Hospital. He remained there in practice for the rest of his life, making only one further journey to Europe in 1673, when he accompanied two English plenipotentiaries to Cologne, where a peace treaty was being negotiated between England, France, and the Netherlands. From 1704, until his death in 1708, he was President of the College of Physicians. He was said to have resembled his father 'in the genteelness of his humour, learning, and manner of practice'. He was esteemed by the aristocracy and became a physician to king Charles II, who knighted his father. The king said that Edward 'was as learned as any of the College, and as well bred as any at court'. Browne published the first report of his travels in 1673; *A brief account of some travels in Hungaria, Servia, Bulgaria, Macedonia, Thessaly, Austria, Styria, Carinthia, Carniola and Friuli*. To an edition published in 1677, he added *An account of several travels through a great part of Germany; I. From Norwich to Colen; II. From Colen to Vienna, with a particular description of that particlar city; III. From Vienna to Hamburg; IV. From Colen to London*; . . . This was reprinted in 1685 in folio and was entitled *A brief account of some Travels in divers parts of Europe, &c., &c.*

Browne sailed off to Rotterdam a year after the end of the second Anglo-Dutch war. He had seen the restoration of the monarchy in 1660 and was at Oxford during those calamitous three years of the Great Plague (1665), the Fire of London (1666), and the humiliating destruction of the fleet at Chatham when the Dutch sailed up the Medway (1667). But they were also the years when the young Isaac Newton at Cambridge was making his momentous discoveries in differential calculus and in the laws of gravity, and when the blind John Milton, in London, was finishing *Paradise Lost*.

On the continent of Europe, France, under Louis XIV, was rising at the expense of Spain and Austria—Holland was in possession of an expanding trading empire—and in central Europe stability was slowly returning after the devastation of the Thirty Years War.

In a note to his readers, Browne said that he was encouraged to publish an account of his journeys as they were living in 'an age, so curious and inquisitive, and withall so industrious, that every day addeth new Informations and Accounts, both of our own country and foreign parts'. Some were to places 'which had been passed by few Englishmen . . . you are not to expect the names of all the places . . . yet divers will you find mentioned, which are not to be found in Mapps; except you have some more exact than any I have met with'. No maps were included

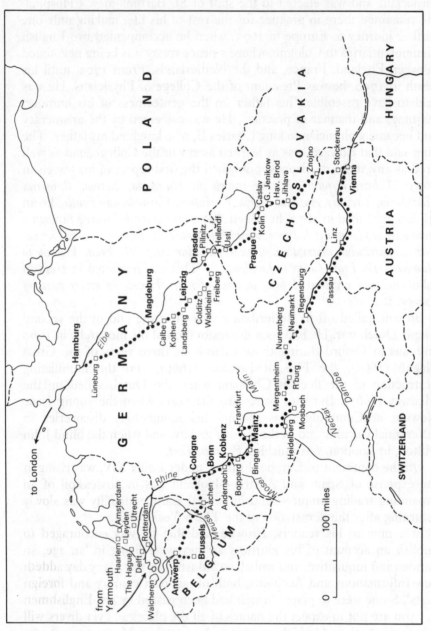

EDWARD BROWNE: JOURNEY TO VIENNA, 1668–9

in his book and he apologized that the few illustrations had been made 'from my own rude draughts and directions'.

I. THE JOURNEY TO VIENNA

He sailed from Yarmouth at 6 p.m. on 14 August in a 55-ton ketch, reaching Rotterdam twenty-four hours later. For the next six weeks he travelled about Holland, by road and boat, before turning south to Belgium, and then east to Cologne, where he arrived on 10 October. He was favourably impressed by the general prosperity in Holland and 'the ease of accommodation for travel by land and water . . . the excellent order and regular course in all things', but said nothing of its inns and what he ate and drank. There were 'good towns', an 'extraordinary neatness', an 'incredible' amount of shipping, an industrious air everywhere, with 'not a beggar in the streets'. He was amazed by what had been accomplished in so small a country.

In Rotterdam he admired the merchants Exchange, the tall houses, and he visited the birthplace of Erasmus. In Delft there was a fine market place, and the tomb of Van Tromp, the Dutch admiral who had defeated the Spanish fleet off the Flemish coast in 1639, and had fought many a battle against the English in the channel, before he was killed there in 1653. But Browne does not mention Leeuwenhoek, the microscopist of Delft, who was busy there at the time examining the capillaries of blood vessels. At The Hague he saw a road running straight through the dunes 'paved by brick for three miles' and lined on each side by four or five rows of trees. He said 'The Hague and Madrid are accounted the greatest villages, or open unwalled places in Europe'.

Leyden, he thought, was one of the neatest towns of Europe, where water flowed in canals in the middle of the tree-lined streets. He saw the physic garden and in the university, founded by William of Orange in 1575, as a reward for the heroic defence the previous year when it was besieged by the Spaniards, he was shown 'many sorts of Optick glasses' and anatomical specimens. Leyden's medical school became very famous in the eighteenth century. In Haarlem there was a hospital for sixty old people, which had a pleasant quadrangle and garden. There was also a hospital for the sick.

Amsterdam was a city 'scarce yielding to any other place in the world'—with fine docks crowded with shipping, warehouses and merchant building, East India Company houses, and a town hall having spacious rooms, marble floors and a richly gilded roof, 'with Atlas and a ten foot copper globe atop'. Yet the whole city was built on marshy ground and rested on a forest of piles, with dozens of bridges and waterways. 'If a man could see all under the City he could hardly behold a greater forest'. For the foundations of one tower, 6334 fir trees were said to have been used. In one of the East India Company houses he saw a copper terrestrial globe, six or seven feet in diameter, which depicted Van Diemen's discoveries in the Far East up to 1642. Trumpets sounded from steeples at six in the morning and in the evening; idleness was not permitted. In a 'house of correction', young men had to labour for their bread. Some sawed Brazil wood and were covered with red dust, others worked in a cistern where they had to pump out the water to keep dry. Young women 'who lived loosely or were taken in the night' worked at domestic chores in another house. There was a mental hospital and also one for orphan children.

In Amsterdam he met some famous men. There was Gerard Blasius, anatomist and physician, who wrote the first important book on the spinal cord in 1666; Frederik Ruysch, professor of anatomy, renowned for his anatomical preparations and preserved bodies with wax injected vessels. They were much praised by Dr Johnson who said Ruysch's corpses glowed 'with the striking lustre and bloom of youth'. Jan Swammerdam demonstrated 'divers of his experiments'. A brilliant microscopist and an entomologist, he pointed out the advantages of the frog for neurophysiological experiments, introducing the nerve-muscle preparation. But to non-medical readers it is the name of 'Old Glawber the Chemist' which will be the most familiar. He was the German chemist, Johann Rudolf Glauber, who had settled in Amsterdam, and made his living by the sale of medicinal preparations, the most notable of which was Glauber's Salt, or sodium nitrate, still used as an aperient. In Utrecht he inspected some 'unicorn horns'—which he explained were twisted horns or 'a long-wreathed tooth' of the narwhal. His father owned one and they had an ancient reputation for protection against poisoning. The Royal Society had examined rhinoceros horn—with negative results—but Browne did not mention this. 'In a high turret' at Dordrecht, cradle of the United Provinces, he dined in a room overlooking the countryside, in which 'our seats moved round the table continually, so as the diversity of the prospect made it more delightful'. The Groote Kerk, there, still has a massive square tower with 365 steps, but it is doubtful if the Reformed Church would have allowed a dining room. It was the seats, and not the room, which revolved, perhaps by windmill power; there are many windmills there although Browne does not actually mention them anywhere in Holland. Dordrecht must have had some tourist-minded businessmen.

He sailed through the islands of Zeeland to Walcheren, where there had been 'a Scots factory' at Veere, 'for 200 years'. This was part of the Scottish wool trade and the local museum is still called De Schotse Huizen (the Scottish Houses). At Flushing, 'one of the first towns which low-country men took from Spain in 1572', he recalled its first governor, Sir Philip Sidney; it was near there he received his fatal wound which is said to have occasioned the well-known words.

Antwerp, then a walled and moated city, he reached by sailing up the Scheldt. The journey to Brussels was also by water, with many locks and five changes of boat. He saw 'the pissing boy' in the townhall square, dined at a fish tavern, but turned back to Antwerp because of plague. 'Three hundred houses were shut up'; garlands with the letters IHS hung on their doors.

From Antwerp he travelled by road to Maastricht and then on to Aachen and Cologne where he arrived on 10 October. He reminds us that Cologne was originally a Roman colony and that for centuries it was an archbishop's See, so it contained many churches and convents and monasteries, as well as its cathedral. But it was also a free imperial city where the territorial rights of the bishops were long contested, with the eventual transfer of the See to Bonn. The archbishop still had two palaces in Cologne but he was not able to reside there for more than three days at a time. The prosperity of the city was based on trade and the quays were filled with long, round-bellied boats from the Low Countries. Its university was founded in 1388, and there were hospitals and dispensaries; the Cologne pharmacopoea was famous.

Here he embarked on a Rhine boat drawn by horses and proceeded to Bonn and Andernach, but finding this tedious, he rode by horse with a German and some friars, as far as Coblenz. There he resumed the river route to Mainz and Frankfurt 'the passage or ford of the Franks'. Whether his boats were horse-drawn all the way is not clear, but he lodged at various villages and towns on the way—Boppard, Rudesheim, Bingen, and Mainz. He reached Frankfurt on about 23 October. He had missed the autumn trade fair—'an extraordinary concourse of people and commodities, especially of books'. The Knights of the Teutonic Order had a house there in which certain criminals could seek temporary sanctuary.

He went by road to Heidelberg, through pleasant country, crossing the Neckar into the town by a covered wooden bridge. He visited the university, 'founded in 1346', saw the townhall clock perform some of its repertoire of entertaining 'divers motions', and admired the 'Great Tun' or carved wooden wine vat in the castle cellar (not the one there today, which dates from 1751). Browne had seen the university's great library of 3500 manuscripts in the Vatican, where it had been sent by Maximilian I of Bavaria in 1623 (coming back to Heidelberg, via Paris, in 1815). He met two Englishmen, belonging to a neighbouring religious community of 100 English, men, women, and children, who called themselves 'Christian Jews'. They had been there since 1661, and their leader was a Mr Poole of Norwich. The next part of his journey took him eastwards across Bavaria, to Nuremberg, and Regensburg on the Danube. He started off on horseback with a German army captain and commented that construction of a waterway between Rhine and Danube had once been started by the emperor Charlemagne in the eighth century. After 'two German miles' he had been defeated by rain, bogs, and 'warlike diversions', but 'it was a noble design' and would have provided communication between the North Sea and the Black Sea.

The Danube boats on which he travelled on to Vienna, were flat-bottomed, broad at both head and stern, and carried 'a chamber built in the middle'. He lodged at nights in places along the river, reaching Passau on 15 November, Linz on the 16th, and Vienna on the 20th. From Regensburg to Vienna, a distance of about 220 miles, took him ten days or so. There were a few dangerous spots, in one of which, below Passau, there were very fast currents, submerged rocks, and a whirlpool. This place was the object of one of his sketches. It was customary there, on safely completing the passage, to pay alms to a monk who came out in a boat from a monastery on the shore.

Vienna

He spent the winter here in lodgings, not actually described, but in apparent comfort and enjoyment. It was 'a healthy place' although 'colic was endemial, very hardly yielding to good medicine'. The Danube froze over, horse-drawn sleighs carried 'ladies in velvet and furs' through the narrow streets, between tall houses often of six to seven storeys, and people walked in the Prater, and drank and listened to music in the inns. There were excellent heating stoves in the latter, in the schools and churches, as well as in the houses. He said that in some parts of Germany 'they lodge and eat in Stoves'. 'Lying between two Feather-beds, with a neat laced sheet spread over', he slept warmly at night. Food supplies were ample—corn, sheep, oxen, boar, hare, rabbit, partridge, pheasant and fish. There was wine, about which he made no comment, and 'some odd dishes' such as guinea-pig, tortoise, and snail. Many nationalities were to be seen, 'all in their proper habits'; German,

French, Italian, Spanish, Polish, Hungarian, Slovakian, Transylvanian, Greek, Tartar, and Turkish. There were ambassadors from Naples, the Vatican, Venice, and many German kingdoms. The ambassador from the Cham of Tartary was there, to confirm a peace; the Tartars were 'a great torment to Eastern Europe . . . carrying off thousands of people to sell to the Turks'.

The city itself stood inside a wall of fortifications with six gates, and 'separated from the suburbs by a fair esplanade'—the Glacis of later days. On top of the steeple of St. Stephens cathedral, with 'its thick-painted glass and tiles of wood', stood the Turkish crescent and star, above a cross. This arrangement was agreed with the Turks during a siege, so that the steeple would be spared bombardment. The Emperor Leopold was a grave and graceful person with 'a long chin and Austrian lip' who was musical and who liked to play church organs. As well as German, he spoke Italian, Spanish, and Latin and was 'a great countenancer of learned men'. Browne became friendly with the emperor's librarian, who allowed him to borrow books from the Imperial Library. The librarian had recommended *Religio Medici* to the emperor and was delighted when he discovered that his English visitor was the author's son. Browne was surprised at the richness of the library, standing 'upon the extreme borders of the learned part of Europe'; it compared well with that of the Bodleian and Vatican. In addition to the thousands of manuscripts and books, there were rooms of 'curiosities' of all kinds—crowns, jewels, carvings, clockworks, and so on. There was a chain of pearls nine yards long, and a knife which intrigued him. It had been swallowed by a peasant near Prague, and removed from his stomach nine months later, in 1602. 'Safely cut out', said Browne, suggesting that the peasant survived.

Over the entrance gate to the Imperial palace, were carved in capital letters, 'the five vowels, AEIOU, whereof the phancies of men make various interpretations'. One was *Austriae est Imperare Orbi Universo*, and another, *Alles Erdreich ist Osterreich Unterthan*—'All the world is subject to Austria'. In the university where there were four national divisions—Austrian, Rhine, Hungarian, and Saxon—'they followed the old beaten way of knowledge; and I met with few who had any good insight into New Philosophy'. He was asked about the Royal Society of London, and he expressed the hope that they would soon 'fall into the ways of experimental philosphy'. He had had similar enquiries in Germany.

In a 'public anatomy' of a beheaded woman, in a theatre holding one hundred, 'the lecture lasted so long that the body was nineteen days unburied'. He actually witnessed two beheadings. In each the victim was seated and he learned that the right hand was first cut off, if there had been treason or 'high crime'. When one head rolled to the ground, a man ran out of the crowd 'with a Pot in his hand and filled it with blood still spouting out of the Neck; he presently drank it off and ran away'. Browne had read that such blood was thought to have medicinal properties and that Celsus had written that epileptics would drink the blood of fallen gladiators.

He visited 'a noble stable of horses' and described the skill of boar hunters, who could tell from the tracks whether the animal was male or female,* young or old, wild or domesticated. 'They chiefly conjecture from their tread or foot, and the casting of their hindfeet out of the track of their forefeet'. He referred to street entertainments, in particular 'One Notable Trick', which reminds one of the peculiar feats which were once so popular, like sword-swallowing and fire-eating.

A man of a middle stature laid down on his back, and a heavy anvil was placed upon his breast, as much as two men could well lift. Then two other men with great hammers laid on until they had given almost an hundred blows, and cut in sunder a great horseshoe of iron, about half an inch thick.

In our day, Houdini explained that the heavier the anvil, the less were the blows felt.

Browne several times mentions the status of the Jews. In Amsterdam they lived 'more handsomely and splendidly than in any other place' and were not required to wear a distinctive dress. In Frankfurt he was told there were 7000 Jews there; there were many in Cologne and Prague. In general they were made to wear 'distinctive habits'—yellow hats in Avignon; taffeta-covered hats in Italy; ruffs, gowns, and capes in Germany. In Vienna, 'They were much distasted by the citizens and tradesmen, and the scholars agree but ill with them'. They had their homes outside the city walls, 'departing each night'. While he was there fighting broke out 'in the Jews Town' when it was invaded by the scholars. Many on both sides were killed and a guard of soldiers was thrown around the place. Browne said that subsequently Jews were banished from Austria, although 'to ingratiate with the Empress, then with child, presented her with a noble silver cradle, but she would not receive it'. Browne regretted this, as he found Jews 'seemed useful unto the place for ready accommodation of any thing, either by sale or exchange . . .'. Jewish physicians were preferred to Christian ones, as

* The Beaver Indians of Alaska can tell whether they are tracking bull or cow from the angle at which urine has hit the snow.

they 'profess skill in urines'. He added that common folk were very credulous about Jewish physicians; they would even believe that 'they had some old Receipts of King Solomon'.

II. JOURNEYS FROM VIENNA

During the spring, summer, and autumn months of 1669 Browne made three journeys from Vienna.

I. The first, of about 300 miles, he entitled *A journey from Komara or Gomora to the minetowns of Hungary and from thence to Vienna*. Komara—now Komaron—is on the Danube, about 120 miles below Vienna, where the river now forms the boundary between Hungary and Czechoslovakia. The mines he visited are in the Carpathian mountains, in the region of Kremnica, now in the southeast part of Czechoslovakia. They had been worked for centuries. Browne said little of his mode of travel or what company he may have had, but most of it must have been on horseback, although he once mentioned an 'hussar who drove the chariot' and also an escort of 'German musketeers in the Contribution Country'.

He went north from Komaron along the river Nitra and then turned eastwards, crossing the river Hron, and heading into the mountains. He went down a silver mine, the largest in the region, called 'Trinity'. It was 70 fathoms deep—420 feet—and he descended it on three long ladders 'almost perpendicular and of about 300 steps'. A large water wheel was used to turn the engines which pumped out the water. He described the processes involved in excavation, pounding and burning the ore, a hundred pounds of which commonly yielded a half to one ounce of silver. In nearby caves and pools there were hot baths, some sulphurous, in common use and greatly valued therapeutically. In a gold mine, 170 fathoms deep—1020 feet—nine to ten miles long, the miners descended, not by ladders, but slung on a leather seat at the end of a cable. Browne also bravely went down this mine—'lowered gently'—and inspected the workings below. He was amazed at the engineering involved in the erection of shafts, tunnels, and galleries, and remained there for some hours. They were all lined with pine-tree trunks and ore was conveyed on small carts called 'Dogs'. Each had four wheels and a centre rail which prevented deviation; 'A little boy will run full speed with three or four hundred pounds of weight of ore or earth before him'. There were air shafts and miners had lamps which went out when there was 'Damp'; fatalities occurred. In the house of a manager of a copper mine, Browne was impressed by the size, detail, and scale of the great

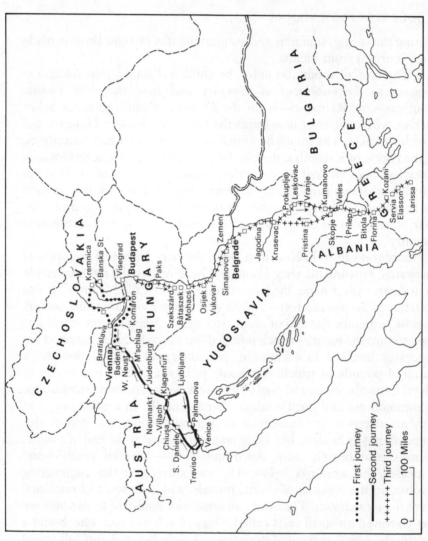

EDWARD BROWNE: JOURNEYS FROM VIENNA IN 1669

First journey

Second journey

+++++ Third journey

0   100 Miles

maps which were used; they provided 'a picture of so fair a subterranean city'.

His route back to Vienna took him across the river Vah, and down to Bratislava (then Pressburg) the capital of Hungary since the Turkish conquest of Budapest in 1541. This was the route taken by Dr Richard Bright in 1815 when he, too, visited the mines of Kremnica.

II. His second tour was *A journey into Styria, Carinthia, Carniola and Friuli*. Carniola was a former crownland of Austria, centred around Ljubljana, now in Yugoslavia; Friuli was the adjacent district at the head of the Adriatic Sea, astride the present boundary of Yugoslavia and Italy. This circuit, around 700 miles, was undertaken in May, June, and July, and again he does not say if he set out in company, or rode in a carriage or on horseback. He passed by way of Baden, 'a pretty, walled town', where he took the baths and was presented with 'a *Gempskugel* which is said to be an excrescence upon the liver of a wild goat of Tirol, and highly cryed up in Germany as a signal remedy against diseases of the liver, malignant fevers and the plague'. From Wiener Neustadt he crossed the Styrian Alps, where the road was so steep that it required 'twenty-four horses or oxen to draw up a cart or coach'. He continued by way of Judenburg* and Neumarkt to St. Veit, where he saw and sketched a fountain basin hewn from a single block of white marble. It measured 'five of my fathoms in circumference'—that is, five lengths of his outstretched arms. In these districts there many goitrous people.

Many here have great throats, some as big as their heads, many are blind, divers dumb, and fools withall; without the town there is an hospital for such as have lost their voice, their wits, or are otherwise oppressed by their great throats . . . the better sort of people which live well, drink wine and good beer, are less subject to them. I saw bigger throats in these parts, than any I had observed in the Alpine part of the Savoy.

The association between feeblemindedness and goitre in Alpine populations was described by several physicians in the seventeenth century, but it was not known whether it was air, water, or food which was responsible. It was not until iodine was discovered early in the nineteenth century, that some alpine waters were found to be deficient in the element. And only in this century was it shown that it was vital for the formation of thyroxine.

Klagenfurt, the capital of Carinthia, was full of soldiers; it was strongly fortified and the Count Commander was very impressed when he learned that Browne knew the Earl Marshal of England—the Earl of Norwich. He learned of 'an old custom there'. A man who was strongly

* 'Jews Town' is still to be seen in modern maps of Austria.

suspected of theft would be hanged; three days later, if he was then judged guilty, his body would be left to rot on the gallows; but if proved innocent, he would then be given a Christian burial.

The road took him southward across the river Drave and over the Karavanke mountains. It was very steep and winding 'with walls turning backwards and forwards with great pains'. It passed through a tunnel, roofed with wood, 156 yards long and 4 yards wide. Carriages could pass in both directions and the road was said to have been kept clear of snow in the winter, as it was the main route between the capitals of Carinthia and Carniola (Ljubljana).

In Ljubljana he met 'a Scotch apothecary', a Mr Tosh, who provided him with much local information. He was intrigued by a nearby lake which emptied in June and refilled in September, through holes in the ground. But the fish in it were in no way unusual. He wondered whether Strabo had seen it. At Idria, there were quicksilver mines where he inspected the furnaces and retorts; in an adjacent castle he saw hundreds of barrels of mercury, and in the visitors' book he noted the names of 'Mr. Evelyn and Dr. Pope'. In the Diary of John Evelyn, I could not find any mention of a visit there, but he may have passed this way on his journeys to and from Italy in 1643–6.

At Palmanova, an historical bulwark against the Turks, he said the fortifications were the finest he had seen anywhere in Europe; there were elaborate bastions and three drawbridges which could be lowered at the touch of an iron; the walls were double and the moat could be flooded. A canal ran from the town to the sea. He went on by felluca to Livenza and Venice, disembarking at the piazza of St. Mark. The Venetian Republic was then in decline 'and were concerned about the Candia siege'. This was in reference to the recent fall of the Venetian city of Heraklion in Crete; it had been besieged by the Turks for two years and 30 000 Venetians were lost. Browne spoke to British sailors who had been there.

Browne did not feel it necessary to write of the well-known sights of Venice. He went to Padua to see some old friends and then turned for home after a short stay. He travelled north through Treviso and Chiusa, over the Julian Alps to Klagenfurt, and then, by the same road he had taken in coming from Vienna. He said that it was 350 miles from Venice to Vienna. He went alone on horseback the whole way, using only one horse. 'It was the quietest journey I ever made.' Of this second journey he said, that as there was little to be observed 'in the common road, I fetched a compass, and came about, passing from place to place, according as remarkable things or curiosities invited.'

III. Browne's third journey—to *Hungaria, Servia, Bulgaria, Macedonia and Thessaly*—was 'hard and unusual, through a good part of European Turkie, and passed by few Englishmen.' It took him, for some 1500 miles, through what now are the countries of Hungary, Yugoslavia, and Greece, in the autumn months of 1669. It had been a hot, dry summer, and there were fevers in this 'new stage of the world, quite different from that of the western countries.'

He went by road to Bratislava, where he saw Turkish prisoners in underground dungeons in the market place, begging through iron bars to passers by. At Komaron, he embarked in a Danube boat which had twenty-four oarsmen, Hungarians rowing on one side and Germans on the other. Before reaching Visegrad, where the Danube turns south, they were met by a Turkish vessel, which towed them to that town. From there he continued down the river to Budapest, where he caught his first glimpse of Turkish women in their 'long breeches and smocks' and covered faces. He was well treated by the Turks, but he noticed that in the streets, foot soldiers resented the presence of horsemen.

From Budapest he continued by road, along the west bank of the Danube, through a flat countryside, to Belgrade. He stayed, presumably with guides and servants, at *Khans* or Caravanserais, the Eastern quadrangular inns with an inner courtyard. They carried their own provisions and prepared their fires and meals in the courtyard. On the way, he saw many gypsies, and droves of cattle wending their way to Vienna, and he spied the occasional Roman ruin or inscription. Oxen drew the ploughs and carts, the latter with spokeless wooden wheels. Bridges were nearly all of wood, and one, over the river Drava, was five miles long, fitted with railings, and a tower every quarter of a mile. 'It was the greatest passage unto Hungary from Servia and the Turkish domains.' On the plains before Simanovci, there were people who lived 'like troglodytes' in small huts half underground, where they 'ran like conies when we passed.' Browne inspected and sketched them and was surprised to find they had partitions, chimneys, and small windows. At Zemen, reaching the Danube again, the final short passage to Belgrade was made on the river.

It was a busy, crowded town, with streets of timber, and many open shops, and merchants' houses. He stayed with an Armenian as they were 'more reasonable than Jews or Greeks.' The large caravanserai there possessed a fountain in its courtyard. There was a castle, a college with turbanned students, and many different public baths. The men were stout, the horses good, and the wine too. 'In Christian hands it might make a flourishing city.'

From Belgrade the way south took him through hilly, and then mountainous country, on horseback and 'in open chariots' drawn by two or three horses abreast. They made good speed, usually covering twenty miles a day, along the west bank of the river Morava. They traversed great woods, where wolves and robbers lurked, with pistols at the ready, and they passed one river 'ninety times in 12 hours.' They went by way of Jagodina, Krusevac, Prokupije, Kumanova, to Veles on the river Vardar, flowing down to the sea at Salonika. Then they climbed into the mountains of Macedonia, by Prilep and Bitola, in sight of Mt Olympus, seventy miles distant. The road was dangerous, with precipices and great overhanging rocks, but with fine views of hillside villages, mosques and Greek monasteries, and many a dead horse by the wayside. At one place there was an aqueduct with 100 arches, and on one hilltop 'an old man with a drum gave notice to passengers on both sides' that there were no roving robbers about. Descending, they came to the town of Servia, where Christians occupied the upper quarter, and Turks the lower. In the plains of Thessaly they were greeted by cotton fields and vineyards.

The journey ended at Larissa on the plain below Olympus and that strategic historical pass between it and the sea. Here, Browne reminds us, many battles were fought in the days of Philip of Macedon, Xerxes, and Alexander. Now it was a great military centre, with fields of tents, and thousands of horses and camels. The bridles and saddles of the horses gleamed brightly in the sun. There were also many Greek merchants and Portuguese Jews; Browne's French and Latin were 'useless.' It was a noisy, hot, and dusty town, yet on Mt Olympus that summer, men had died of the cold. The town had three mosques and eighteen churches. The Sultan was 'inclined to fatness', but a strong, hard rider, fond of hunting with the hawk in the hills. Footmen and horsemen, with banners and music, frequently accompanied him. They were a warlike race, revengeful and cruel. The local people usually hid from the Sultan when he appeared, although he wished to be friendly.

Many kinds of fruit and vegetables grew in the surrounding countryside. There were groves of olive, fig, and lemon trees; vineyards, fields of water melon, tobacco and sesame, garlic, and large onions. There was a gourd-like fruit, 'between a melon and a cucumber', called a 'Melanzan', which Browne particularly enjoyed. When the seed was cut away from the centre, it could be filled with sausage meat and then boiled.

He found the Turks polite, and good guides. They shaved their heads, leaving only a lock of hair on the crown. Croats cut their hair on only one side of the head; Hungarians shaved it all 'except for the foretop'; the Polanders (Polish) cut theirs short; the Franks wore their hair long 'as with us'; Greeks shaved a bare area on the crown, but their priests did not cut their hair at all. The Turks told him that the Russian was best at the oar, the Georgian made a good counsellor, and the Albanian a good courtier. Turks spoke many languages and distrusted maps. Careful about their toilet, 'When they go the house of office, they carry a pitcher of water with them; they affect privacy when they make water, which they perform resting on one knee, and stretching out the other leg.' But they were not content with their empire. Browne heard them say that they should get beyond Hungary and lay siege again to Vienna. This they did, of course, in 1683, only to be driven back once more.

As he made his preparations for returning to Vienna, which he did by more or less the same route, he mused that in all probability, the 'same habits, manners and course of life' which he had seen in these lands, would also be found in all Asia, 'even unto China.'

III. VIENNA TO HAMBURG

Browne returned home, by stage-coaches, through Czechoslovakia and Germany, by way of Prague, Dresden, Freiburg, Leipzig, Magdeburg, and Hamburg. He set out in mid-November and arrived in England at the end of December, having been away for seventeen months. He said that the stage from Vienna to Prague, through the hills and forests of Moravia and Bohemia—a distance of about 200 miles—normally took eight days in winter and six in summer. En route he made particular enquiries about the sprite called 'Ribensal', which was said to infest the country. It haunted the hills and woods and mines, singing and playing on bagpipes, dressing up sometimes as a monk, and generally tormenting folk. Little had been heard of him for the previous twelve years, but Browne's inquisitiveness probably reflected the superstitious streak in his mind. It was only five years earlier that his father had given evidence at a trial of two witches at Norwich. He was a witness for the prosecution and they were hanged.

At Prague, the university had fewer students than in the days of John Huss, when he had been rector. The great bridge across the river Vltava had sixteen arches and a tower at each end; it led the way up to the castle and cathedral on the Hradcany hill, with its fine views. High German was spoken here, and Jews flourished, especially in the jewelry trade. Browne purchased some topazes. He could not proceed by boat down the river to the Elbe (presumably it was frozen) and went by road. It was rough in parts, made up of 'trees laid side by side'. But, as they got into Saxony, the countryside began to look gentler and more cultivated than the 'forests and rocks of Bohemia.'

Dresden was a fine place—prosperous-looking and well fortified—and possessing a palace for the Elector, a museum, a library and even a zoo 'the garden of the Hunting House.' Here he made a sketch to illustrate how well the fifteen bears were catered for; there were also lions and tigers. The galleried and decorated horse stables were 'extraordinary noble.' 'Each horse eats out of a rack of iron, and a manger of copper; and on a pillar by him, his comb, bridle and saddle.' In the library and museums he saw many fine mathematical instruments and charts, intricate clockwork machines for toys and instruments—a cuckoo which sang, a ship which sailed, an old woman who walked, a centaur which ran, and 'a crab creepeth upon a table so well as to amaze and delight.' In the 'chamber of curiosities' there were hundreds of objects displayed; fowls made out of mother of pearl, gold drinking cups fashioned in the shape of dragons or elephants; a cherry stone on which had been carved one hundred-and-twenty-one heads; a crystal cabinet sold by Oliver Cromwell; King Charles II of England on horseback, in iron; figures of fish in various stones and so on. Browne was amazed by the display of skill and workmanship on the part of joiners, turners, smiths, barbers, and surgeons. Lutheran women he noted wore white, not black, when in mourning. And it was they, and not the men, who said grace at meals.

At Freiburg he saw something of the silver, gold, and lead mines, sketching some miners and observing that 'the greatest trouble they have is by dust, which spoileth their lungs and stomach, and frets their skin.' On the road to Leipzig, there was a place called 'Goldick', which we know as Colditz.

Leipzig was 'a rich trading city', famous for its fairs, and to whose university thousands of students flocked on leaving Prague in Huss's day. It had the 'fairest Lutheran church', St. Nicholas, in all Germany. Browne did not mention the Thomaskirche which was there, and later to be memorable for its association with J. Sebastian Bach. As in Dresden, there was evidence of learning as well as trade. 'The burgomaster had five fair daughters brought up in commendable ways, schooled in Holland and fluent "in divers languages".' In another 'chamber of rarities' was displayed 'the garter of an English bride' with an accompanying explanation that 'it was the fashion in England for the brideman (the best man) to take it off and wear it in his hat.' This seemed strange to the Germans, but Browne vouched for it, saying that 'I had often done it myself.'

At Magdeburg, on the Elbe, he stayed at the house of an old man who was there when the city was sacked and burned, and most of its people were butchered by Count Tilly's soldiers in 1631. Here also, he said, that tournaments were first held in Germany, in the year 635. They are generally regarded as having been started in France, in the tenth century. But Browne said that Henry the 'Fowler', Duke of Saxony and King of Germany, began it to increase proficiency in arms. Henry I died in 936, so Browne had got his date wrong. However, he was knowledgeable about horsemanship, and learned about the customs and rules concerning tournaments there. Certain people were debarred from taking any part—bastards, cowards, traitors, murderers and heretics, oppressors of widows and orphans, and all those who 'had given offence to ladies by word or deed'. Medieval chivalry was making its bow.

'The winter growing on', Browne felt he had to make haste to Hamburg. He went there by stage-coach in four days, a distance of some 120 miles, through a barren-looking country side of heath and winds and few inns. Hamburg was 'full of strangers and merchants of every country . . . and aboundeth in shipping'. The English Company was flourishing and had 'good privileges'. 'Ships come laden with cloth to the value of an hundred thousand pounds sterling.' In Hamburg they were happiest when the princes of Europe were not at war.

Germany had impressed him. It profited from its four great waterways—the Danube, Rhine, Elbe, and Oder—and had no less than sixty-six imperial free cities. There were great mines and hundreds of workshops where 'singular artificers and industrious workmen' were employed. The people were 'plain-dealing and trusty', the traveller 'more secure' than in many other countries, and the houses were well-built and warm and clean. Germans were nevertheless 'naturally martial' and regiments of them were to be found in most European armies. But Germany 'was not exhausted by the Sea, nor by colonies sent forth, or by the peopling of American countries.' Following the devastation of the plague and the Thirty Years War, they had made a striking recovery; 'the effects were scarcely discernible'. Indeed, said Browne, 'Germany is a great Hive of Men'.

He sailed from Hamburg on 10 December but what with a calm, contrary winds, and the eventual storm off the coast of Kent, he did not put his foot ashore, after anchoring 'in Margaret Road', until 'Christmas Morning (praised be God)'.

3

John Bell's Travels in Russia and Asia
1715-1737

JOHN BELL (1691–1780), the author of *Travels from St. Petersburg in Russia to various parts of Asia in 1716, 1719, 1722 &c*, published in Glasgow in 1763, was the son of Patrick Bell of Antermony, and was born on the paternal estate. Both the Dictionary of National Biography and Robert Chambers's *A biographical dictionary of eminent Scotsmen, 1835*, state that Bell had some medical education. Chambers said that 'after receiving a classical education he turned his attention to the study of medicine. On passing physician he determined to visit foreign countries . . .'. The *DNB* stated that 'No details of his education are extant, but it is stated that, after obtaining the degree of doctor of medicine, he determined to visit foreign countries'. Bell himself wrote, in the opening sentence of the preface to his book, that 'In my youth I had a strong desire of seeing foreign parts' and to satisfy such inclinations he secured letters of reference to Dr. Areskine, chief physician and privy-counsellor to the Czar Peter I in St. Petersburg. As it happened, Dr Areskine had been asked to recommend 'someone with a knowledge of physic and surgery' to serve on an embassy which the Czar was sending to Persia. Bell said that 'As I had employed some part of my time in those studies, the Doctor recommended me . . . and also to the College of Foreign Affairs at St. Petersburg, by whom I was engaged in the service of Peter the First.' This was in 1714, when he was twenty-three years of age. Bell makes no other reference to his medical studies and I have not been able to discover anything about them. A John Bell features in the lists of arts students at Glasgow University in 1710–12 and we know there was little organized medical education there before 1730.

His *Travels*, written forty-eight years after setting out on the first of his journeys, were based on diaries. Apparently he used to entertain his friends with stories about them, and was persuaded 'to throw his notes in to some sort of narrative', by the Earl of Granville. Bell had some difficulty in obtaining literary advice, from a Scottish historian and also from an Aberdeen professor, but it was suggested that Gulliver's Travels should serve as a model guide. Bell describes, with one map, four journeys he took from St. Petersburg. I. The first was to Isfahan, Persia, 1715–18; II. The second was to Peking, China, 1719–22; III. The third, to Persia with the Czar's army in 1722; IV. The fourth to Constantinople, Turkey, 1737. Bell does not say how long he lived in Russia, but he seems to have revisited Scotland in 1723 and to have married a Russian lady, 'Mary Peters', in 1746. He then apparently retired to his estate in Scotland, 'enjoying the society of his friends', until his death on 1 July 1780, in his eighty-ninth year.

When young Bell arrived in St. Petersburg in 1714, Czar Peter the First was forty-two years of age, at war with Sweden, creating the first Russian Navy, and building his beloved city on the Neva. He had travelled in Europe and was determined to transform Muscovy into a modern European power. He was exceptionally tall—six feet seven inches—possessed of extraordinary energy, but subject to frightful rages, and an epileptic. He suffered from convulsions since childhood—mainly affecting the left side of his face, neck, and left upper limb. In some of them he became unconscious. This form of focal epilepsy could have been a consequence of some childhood infection, but it was certainly aggravated by excessive drinking when he became an adult. Bouts of restlessness, maniacal activity, orgies, and acts of violence have all been well documented. His personality disorder, his behaviour, and his epilepsy could all be attributed to a brain lesion. Today, he would probably have had neurosurgical treatment.

Bell never mentioned the Czar's epilepsy, nor did he ever say that he had attended him medically. He devoted four pages to comment on his appearance, character and behaviour, and stressed that most of the stories about him were groundless. He first saw him when he came aboard the ship on which Bell was sailing to St. Petersburg in October 1714. He was accompanied by Dr Areskine, who acted as English interpretor. Bell noted nothing untoward; the Czar ate some bread and cheese, drank a glass of ale, and went back ashore. Bell next saw him that winter when he was living with an English ship-builder in the Czar's employ. 'One morning, before daylight, my servant came and told me that the Czar was at the door. I got up and saw him walking up and down the yard, the weather being severely cold and frosty, without any one to attend him.' The Czar discussed some matter about a ship being built, and then left. A bizarre incident, to say the least.

In 1722, in the Astrakhan camp, Bell shared a tent with the physician

who succeeded Dr Areskine. The latter died in 1717. The chief
physician's name was Blumentrost, and for two months their tent was
next to that of the Czar's. Bell noted nothing unusual. He said the Czar
was always sober and abstemious, never vicious or cruel, but he did
admit that perhaps any failing he had 'arose from his inclination to the
fair sex'. Bell had probably left the camp before the Czar became ill with
one of his bouts of strangury and urinary infection. In the remaining two
years before his death he had recurrent urinary obstruction, he was
catheterized, a large calculus was passed, and in the end there were
repeated convulsions.

Bell's portrait of the Czar is not one which has been corroborated by
history.

I. LENINGRAD TO ISFAHAN

This journey began in July 1715 on his appointment as physician to an
embassy which the Czar was sending to Isfahan, then the capital city of
Persia. They travelled first to Moscow, then by river to Gorky and down
the Volga as far as Kazan, where they spent the winter and spring. In
June 1716 they sailed down the Volga, reaching Kuybyshev (Samara) on
20 June, Saratov on 25 June, Stalingrad on 7 July, and Astrakhan, where
the Volga enters the Caspian Sea, on 13 July.

Leaving Astrakhan in a fleet of five vessels on 5 August, they sailed
down the west coast of the sea, past Derbent, to a place called
'Niezabatt', 'two days journey east', arriving there on 30 August.
Niezabatt possessed neither harbour nor creek and I have not been able
to locate it exactly. From there, they journeyed overland, crossing the
eastern end of the Caucasus range of mountains, reaching Tabriz on 27
December, and Isfahan on 14 March 1717.

They remained there until the following September, returning north
by a route which took them east of Tabriz, to Shemakha, in the
Caucasus, where they arrived on 12 December. Here they remained
until the following June, when they sailed back to Astrakhan, from where
they journeyed once more on the Volga, as far as Saratov. From there
they went by road to Moscow and Leningrad, arriving there on 30
December 1718. They had been away for three and a half years.

The ambassador's party comprised about 140; 13 staff, a troop of 25
dragoons, and a hundred or so others—footmen, valets, tailors,
carpenters, smiths, together with 'a band of music, consisting of
trumpets, kettle drums, violins, hautboys &c . . .' They traversed
mountain and desert and frozen land and rivers. They crossed turbulent

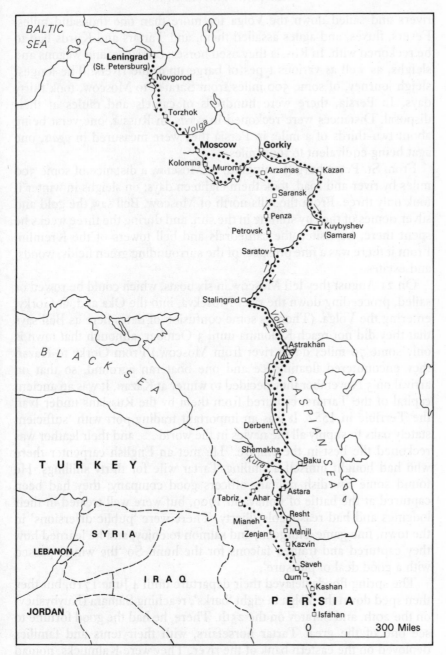

JOHN BELL IN RUSSIA: FIRST JOURNEY, LENINGRAD TO ISFAHAN, JULY
1715–DECEMBER 1718

rivers and sailed down the Volga for more than one thousand miles. Fevers, fluxes, and agues assailed them, and Tartars and Kurds had to be reckoned with. In Russia they used horses, carriages, and wagons and sleighs, as well as various types of barge upon the rivers. The longest sleigh journey, of some 500 miles from Saratov to Moscow, took thirty days. In Persia, there were hundreds of camels and mules at their disposal. Distances were reckoned in *versts*, in Russia, one verst being about two-thirds of a mile; in Persia they were measured in *agats*, one agat being equivalent to four miles.

From St. Petersburg (Leningrad) to Moscow, a distance of some 500 miles by river and road, took them eighteen days; on sleighs in winter it took only three. From the hills north of Moscow, Bell saw the gold and silver domes of the city shining in the sun, and during the three weeks he spent there, he visited the cathedrals and bell towers of the Kremlin. From it there was a fine prospect of the surrounding green fields, woods, and estates.

On 21 August they left Moscow in six boats, which could be rowed or sailed, proceeding down the river Mosckva, into the Oka and, at Gorky, entering the Volga. (There is some confusion of dates here as Bell says that they did not reach Kolomna until 3 October, although that town is only some 70 miles down river from Moscow.) From Gorky to Kazan they encountered floating ice and one boat ran aground, so that on arrival on 5 November they decided to winter at Kazan. It was an ancient capital of the Tartars, captured from them by the Russians under Ivan the Terrible in 1552. It was an important trading port with 'sufficient stately oaks to supply all the navies in the world . . . and their leather was reckoned the best in the empire.' He met an English carpenter there who had bought himself a smiling Tartar wife for thirty shillings. He found some Swedish military officers good company; they had been captured at the battle of Poltava in 1709, but were well treated in their lodgings and had reasonable liberty. There were 'public diversions' in the town, fine game, sturgeon, and salmon to enjoy, and he learned how they captured and trained falcons for the hunt. So 'the winter passed with a good deal of pleasure'.

The spring floods delayed their departure until 4 June 1716, but they then sped down the Volga in eight 'barks', reaching Samara (Kuybyshev) on the 20th, and Saratov on the 25th. There, he had the good fortune to see one of the great Tartar horsefairs, with their tents and families deployed on the eastern bank of the river. They were Kalmucks, nomad Mongolians of the Buddhist faith, who had migrated from the East with their animals in the sixteenth century, eventually reaching the Volga.

Bell was full of praise for their hardiness and spirit, the structure and simplicity of their felt tents which could be erected so quickly and proved so warm. A camel could carry six of them. (Later in the eighteenth century, fearing oppression, they returned east in a disastrous general exodus.)

Near Czaritza (Stalingrad), Bell met an Englishman in charge of construction of a canal intended to link the Volga with the Don, only 35 miles away. But it proved too difficult and the project was abandoned, though it would have linked the Volga with the Black Sea, and reminding us of Dr Edward Browne's comments about Charlemagne's effort to build a canal between the Rhine and the Danube.

Astrakhan, on the Volga delta, another city captured from the Tartars in the sixteenth century, was reached on 13 July. It was a hot and dusty place, surrounded by desert, but with irrigated fields where fruits and vines flourished, and an important trading centre which had become militarily strategic in Peter the Great's campaign against Persia. The skin of the newborn Persian lamb, 'astrakhan', is named after the town. Bell mentions how he had read that 'some grave German authors' alleged that 'Tartarian lamb' was actually a shrub which was capable of partaking of animal, as well as vegetable life. He walked many a mile looking for such shrubs, and although there were some, around which everything had gone, he concluded that it was all a ridiculous fable. In the city, one day, he was struck by the 'extraordinary beauty' of a Tartar lady riding astride an ox, which she guided with a bridle strung through a ring in his nose.

Three weeks after their arrival in Astrakhan they embarked on five vessels, three of them armed with cannon, on the voyage down the Caspian Sea. It actually took them twenty-five days, but twenty of them were spent in a dead calm, in this tideless sea, out of sight of land, and seeing only one other vessel in the meantime. Landing on a beach below Derbent, in high wind and surf, a secretary who was carried ashore on a sailor's back, got lost in some woods. He spent a night in a tree, with howling jackals circling around, and 'scarce ever recovered his former sagacity and soundness of mind'. While camped on the shore, waiting for camels, mules, and provisions, Bell met two Jesuits from India, *en route* for Rome. They were allowed to sail to Astrakhan on one of the boats. Meanwhile, there was fever and sickness in the camp, few were able to dine at the ambassador's table, and several men died. Armed guards were posted, as robbers from the mountains were rumoured to be approaching.

They were glad to raise camp on 18 September and form their

caravan of animals and wagons for the trek to Shemakha, the capital of
the khan or province of Shirvan. Escorted by Persian soldiers, they
reached their destination, a hundred miles inland, on the 27th. Here,
the air was better, although the poor secretary died. They were able to
stroll in the hills, hunt for fowl and hare, and sample the local wines
which Christians kept cool in great jars beneath their gardens. The
mullahs called from the mosques at noon, and from one particular tower
on a hill, at sunrise and sunset, 'came a concert of music, composed of
large trumpets, drums and hautboys which made a dreadful sound'. It
was said to have been a custom from the time of Alexander the Great.
Most of the town's people were Persians, but there were considerable
numbers of Georgians and Armenians. Trade in raw silk was important,
most of it going to English and Dutch factories in Isfahan, and thence to
Aleppo.

The next stage of their march—from Shemakha to Tabriz—involved
crossing the plain of Kurdistan and the river Kura, and winding their
way through the hills and mountains at the eastern end of the Caucasus
range. Commonly taking ten days, with 160 camels and 200 horses and
mules, they actually took twenty-three. Bell recalled that Xenophon had
experience of the warlike Kurds, and they still possessed the finest
horses in Persia. Meeting a Persian hunting party, with greyhounds and
falcons, he was shown how the latter were taught to hover about the
head of an antelope, retarding its flight so that the less swift greyhounds
could catch it. A dead antelope was skinned and stuffed. Food was
placed between its horns and the falcons fed from it. In a similar manner
the birds were taught to attack wolves and foxes. The river Kura was
crossed on a bridge of boats, and in the mountain villages they were
poorly received and forced to spend their nights in cold tents. On high
mountain passes Bell hoped to catch a glimpse of Mt Ararat, a hundred
or so miles to the west, but he was disappointed.

They lingered for a month at Tabriz, in the province of Azerbaijan,
but there was little to see except some mosques, for everywhere there
were signs of destruction and agricultural decay. It had been devastated
by wars and earthquakes, and had only been won back (temporarily)
from the Turks, after a century of occupation. In the surrounding,
rainless countryside, irrigation ways had been only partially restored but
fruits, rice, grain, and cotton were then growing, and raw silk and
carpets still manufactured.

Snow and cold winds made much of their final three week march to
Isfahan very slow and arduous. Snowblindness, exhaustion, and fighting
camels, enforced halts and delays, but as they made their way south, the

going became easier. Reaching Saveh, and then the holy city of Qum, they were greeted with trees in bloom, fine orchards, and large, accommodating caravanserais. At Qum, Bell saw the largest of pomegranates.

At Kashan, the last town of note before Isfahan, Bell heard all about the venomous black scorpion and the dangerous tarantula. One of the latter fell on his hand one night as he was going to bed, but it did no harm. A person poisoned by a tarantula would be put into a cradle suspended by ropes at each of four corners. The ropes were then tightly twisted together and suddenly released. The cradle spun around and the patient would vomit—a sort of therapeutic vertigo. Three days before Isfahan, the Shah sent them a gift of richly accoutred horses, with a couple of lions for display. The lions were let loose on a goat in a courtyard, but attacked some of the Russians instead. Fortunately, only the lion keeper was wounded, and but lightly. The processional entry on horseback into Isfahan on 14 March 1717, was meant to be an imposing one—in full dress, swords drawn, band playing, and all their horses in 'sumptuous trappings'. Bell listed the 'Order of Entry' and a colourful parade they must have made, what with stewards, pages, footmen, and dragoons—not to mention 'Two hey-dukes in Hungarian habits'. The streets and housetops were crowded with spectators and it was rumoured that 'the Sophy himself was at a window *incognito*, with some of his ladies'. They were provided with a palace in the city and no doubt settled down to rest and enjoyment, after their journey of twenty months.

Their stay lasted nearly six months, from March to September 1717. With a pleasant climate and altitude, fertile soil and abundant water for irrigation, it had been chosen as the capital of Persia in the sixteenth century. Shah Abbas I transferred his seat from Kazvin, built palaces and mosques, and invited trade. Bell said it was still 'populous and extensive', but we know that it was already in decline and that before the century was out and as a result of Afghan invasion, its importance diminished. There was a splendid, long, wide, tree-lined avenue, flanked by palaces, administrative buildings, mosques, and colleges, leading to an imposing square or *maidan*. There were gardens and fountains, three fine stone bridges over a river, an immense covered bazaar, and beyond, flat watered fields where crops and fruits flourished. The houses were built of brick hardened by the sun. The streets were not paved, and the inhabitants were accustomed to sit on carpets sipping their coffee and smoking their pipes, in the shade of the trees. Gusts of hot wind sometimes disturbed this tranquil scene. There were Catholic convents and Armenian churches in the suburbs.

Seven weeks were to pass before the Russian ambassador was summoned to one of the seven royal palaces. His suite processed across the maidan, beneath the arched Aali Kapu, or 'God's Gate', into a courtyard where they had to sit for two hours, watching a parade which included an elephant and lions. Then, they were conducted through another arched gateway into a spacious garden some hundreds of yards square, where they admired lines of richly caparisoned horses, with the ambassador receiving obeisance as he passed, even from the elephant and two lions. The elephant bent one fore-limb and the lions 'couched'. The pillared audience chamber stood at the far end of this garden, behind banks of flowers and playing fountains. Bell, with the ambassador and five others, were invited to ascend the marble steps into the pavilion. It was shaded with coloured canvas and had a magnificent arched ceiling, set with mirrors, and with walls adorned with silk carpets, and from which hung branches of foliage made of silver and gold. On a raised couch sat the Shah, a man of 'pleasing open countenance, with a short black beard', whom Bell judged to be about thirty years of age. Letters, gifts, and compliments were exchanged through interpreters and aides, music was played, and after some hours they sat down to dishes of rice, fowl, and lamb, served on gold and china plates, which they ate with their fingers, using wafers of wheat bread as napkins. Bell was disappointed that there were no dancing girls or wine. They drank only sherbet and iced-water. He learned that the ice, which was daily sold in the streets, came from the neighbouring hills. When there was a winter frost, men would set out and water certain slopes, storing the ensuing blocks of ice, in nearby caves, for summer use.

There were other auditions and receptions in which he enjoyed watching tumblers, jugglers, and puppets, dinners at the English and Dutch factories, and trips into the surrounding countryside. There were visitors who passed through—a Dutch governor from Batavia, with presents and six elephants for the Shah, and Christian missionaries from India and Ethiopia. The physician-in-chief knew nothing of European medicine, and enquired about the properties of tea, of which he was also ignorant.

Bell noted that the city was open and defenceless, administration lax, and the military quite untrained. While he was there, fighting had broken out with the Afghans in Kandahar, which had been Persian until 1709. Isfahan itself, though still nominally a capital, declined in importance for the rest of the eighteenth century, and not to the surprise of Bell, writing four decades later. He concluded that the Persians knew little of their ancient history, or of the world itself, and the absurd pomposity of some of the Shah's titles he found most amusing. The one he liked best was that 'The greatest Kings of the earth may think it an honour to drink out of his horses footsteps'.

When they left Isfahan on 1 September, they were laden with gifts of silk carpets, gold, and silver, but one wonders what happened to the elephant, the two lions, the leopard, the monkeys and exotic birds which also accompanied them. The horses would manage and we last hear of the elephant when he was wounded in an attack by tribesmen on the shores of the Caspian. The party returned north to Shemakha, where they wintered, by a route east of Tabriz. Plague had killed many, 70 000 in the province of Shirvan, he learned; they lost 22 of their members. But they sailed to Astrakhan in June, and in five weeks travelled up the Volga to Saratov. From their they set off across country to Moscow, by sleigh, travelling over five-hundred miles in thirty days, and finally reaching St. Petersburg on 30 December 1718—'a city so changed that I could scarcely imagine myself in the same place'.

II. LENINGRAD TO PEKING

After his return from Isfahan, Bell spent eighteen months in St. Petersburg, 'with much satisfaction', before setting out as physician to another embassy, this time, to Peking. He was away for thirty months—from July 1719 until January 1722. There were sixty in the party which sailed once more down the Moscva, Oka, and Volga to Kazan, where the overland journey began. They spent a month there, making their preparations, and left on 28 November for Molotov, travelling through vast forests by sleigh and crossing the frozen river Kama. This stage took eleven days—about 250 miles. At Molotov, famous for its salt mines, Bell saw the huge, single-masted barges— 'longer and broader than a first class English man-o-war'—which were used for transportation of the salt. Each vessel was manned by six to eight hundred men; 40 or 50 men were employed on the rudder alone, itself nearly as long as the barge. When necessary the barges were towed by these men from the banks. Here also there were asbestos mines.

Leaving Molotov on 10 December, they crossed the Ural mountains, where, Bell estimated, they were some forty miles wide, running north to south. Entering Siberia, they proceeded along the banks of the rivers Tura and Tobol, to the city of Tobolsk, arriving on 16 December. It was an important garrison and trading centre, lying in a flat, densely-wooded landscape, where the Tartars proved reliable and honest—and where travel was safe. Fowl, game, and fish were abundant, while in the forests

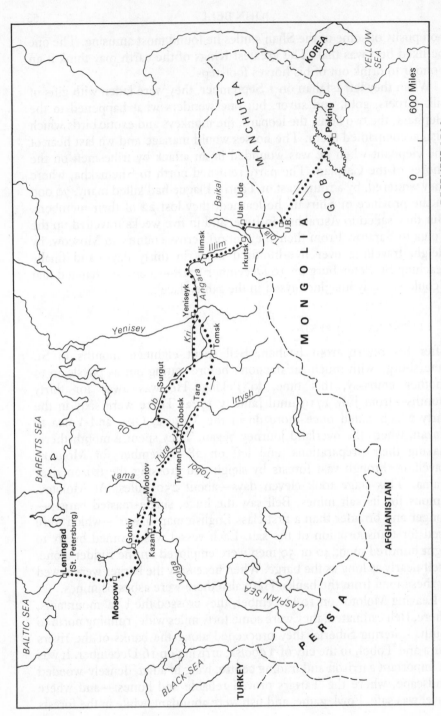

JOHN BELL IN RUSSIA: SECOND JOURNEY, LENINGRAD TO PEKING, JULY 1719–DECEMBER 1722

there were bears, wolves, elk, and reindeer to be hunted. At Tobolsk the river Irtysh joined the Tobol, flowing north to the river Ob and the Arctic Sea.

Now, joined by a party of 25 dragoons, they went down the banks of the Irtysh, staying each night in Tartar villages, for some 330 miles, to the town of Tara, which they reached in seven days. The village huts had one or two clean rooms, a single, low, large bench-type bed covered in furs and rugs, and a window of 'ice-sheet'. Two sheets would last the winter. From Tara, their way lay across a barren, marshy plain, for seventeen days, and across the frozen river Ob, to the city of Tomsk, where they arrived on 4 February. Here Bell saw many Tartar grave-mounds and learned that they often contained gold and silver ornamented swords, bridles, and saddles of ancient warriors. Tobolsk citizens sallied out on summer days to search these graves. Furs from sable, fox, ermine, and squirrel were the major trading commodities, and in the woods there were also said to be species of wild bull and ox—Urus and Bubul. Fish were lured to holes in the ice with fires, and Bell succeeded in the art of spearing them. Cossacks displayed their horsemanship, 'splitting a pole into shivers' with bow and arrow, while at full gallop.

Six of the next fourteen days journey to the town of Yeniseyk, were spent on sleighs on the frozen river Chulym, where they met 'neither house nor inhabitant'. At night they lit large fires on the river bank—'in the space of a minute, the fire mounts to the top of a tree'. The local Tartars were poor, miserable beings, 'with a barbarous language'. After a week's rest at Yeniseyk, they travelled for eleven days on the ice of the Angara river, to the town of Ilimsk. They passed great flocks of five to six hundred hares, travelling westwards along the river banks. Clad in furs, and on snow-shoes, the Tartars here were wholly nomadic, hunting with bow and arrow and reminding Bell of what he had read about Canadian eskimoes, to whom he thought they must be allied. Smallpox had recently decimated them.

Leaving Ilimsk on 12 March, they resumed their sleigh journey down the frozen Angara for several days, then, as the snows were melting, they had to take to their horses and wagons for the remainder of their trek to Irkutsk. 'In the space of a few days we had passed from a cold winter to a warm spring.' Irkutsk, where they arrived on 18 March, was a garrison town near the north shore of the Western end of Lake Baikal, and another important trading and customs post for traffic to and from China. There were some 2000 wooden houses; the local Tartars lived in tents, wore sheepskin garments, tending large herds of cattle and flocks of sheep—but never tilling the ground like the Russian settlers around them.

They had to wait two months at Irkutsk for the ice on Lake Baikal to melt sufficiently; they could have crossed on horseback, but not with their baggage. The lake was some fifty miles wide and three hundred long, Bell estimated; its shores were rocky in parts and storms were frequent. Their crossing by boats, on 15 May, took them a day and a night to reach the mouth of the river Selenga on the south shore. Even then, they encountered ice which they were able to walk on. They sailed or towed their boats up the river towards the towns of Ulan Ude and Kyakhta, through pleasant fertile land, but, tormented by mosquitoes and irked by their slow progress, the staff turned to horses and rode on ahead, making camp on 29 May at a small place of two hundred houses on the banks of the Selenga, near the Chinese border. The river there was 'at least twice the breadth of the river Thames'. Once more, they had to halt for two months, while emissaries went to and fro, from Ulan Bator, the holy city of the Mongols, and from Peking. Precise intentions, letters of information, and credentials had to be submitted to the Emperor of China, before anyone was allowed to set foot in his territories. Most of Bell's time was spent in learning about the Mongols, their mode of living and customs. He enjoyed their company, hunted with them, and also with Cossack troops. The spacious, wooded countryside, with its lakes and large rivers, reminded him of what he had read about the English colonies of America—'particularly the inland parts of Pennsylvania and Maryland'. The lands he had passed through were large enough for 'several European nations', and Mongols would do 'very well for neighbours'.

He met an eighty-year old Tartar chief, so merry and vigorous, on foot or on horse, that one of the rather stout members of the Russian staff enquired how he kept himself so fit and lean. 'Eat less and work more', came the reply; and Bell thought how old Hippocrates would have approved. There was also a seventy-year old fakir from India, on a pilgrimage to the Dalai Lama of Tibet. he had been walking across mountains for a year and pointed out some errors on Bell's maps.

At last, permission to move on through Mongolia to China, was obtained, and on 9 September, they started with their horses, camels, wagons and escorts on their last long march. But some Russian women had to remain behind; no European woman had yet entered China. Through plains and hills covered with a high grass,the caravan made its way, crossing the river Tola on 1 October and then entering the desert. They did not come in sight of the Great Wall until 2 November, when they saw it 'running along the tops of the mountains forty miles away'. Since the crossing of the Tola, Bell wrote, 'we had neither seen river, tree, bush nor mountain'. For 28 days they went from well to well, 'not halting for a single day'.

Their guides directed them to a pass through the mountains; they visited and had tea in a hillside monastery, and spent a comfortable night in a village, where everything was clean and warm. Arriving at the Great Wall on 5 November, they were escorted through a great gate which was closed every night and guarded by 1000 soldiers.

At Wanchuan, their first Chinese city, they dined with the commandant on roast pig, mutton, and fowl, eating with their fingers and 'ivory pins', and drinking tea and arrack. There was strange music from strange wind instruments, and dancing which was only 'a kind of gesticulation and ridiculous posturing'. That night there was a great fall of snow. From there to Peking took them another twelve days across treeless but cultivated country, with long straight roads and signal towers every few miles. Each night they were hospitably cared for; cleanliness, orderliness, and quietness prevailed. There were more giant walls on hilltops, square towers and rocky slopes. At one village they saw a quail-fight, but the game little birds were always separated before serious harm was done. Cock-fighting also took place but it was considered more vulgar.

On the morning of the 18 November, they formed up in procession, and, led by a mandarin with 500 Chinese horsemen, they marched for two hours to the great north gate of the city of Peking. Then, for two more hours they continued down a long, straight road, lined with people gazing with wide-eyes at the white men. At the centre of the city they came to the Russian House where they were to be quartered. It was enclosed by a high brick wall, and there were three courtyards and three single-storeyed groups of buildings, for soldiers, servants, and embassy staff. At ten that night the outer gate was closed, locked and 'sealed with the Emperor's seal' a procedure which caused the Russian ambassador successfully to protest about the following morning.

Peking

The eighty-year old Emperor K'ang-hsi had been on the throne since childhood, following the downfall of the Ming Dynasty and the rise of the militant Manchus. Bell found him sprightly, courteous, and tolerant to the Christians and their missionary endeavours. He was a patron of learning and the arts. There were many ceremonial audiences, banquets and entertainments, and Bell was impressed by the orderliness and calm which prevailed. There was 'never the least noise, hurry or confusion' and no attempt was made to excite wonder or awe in the visitors, as had been the intention at the Persian court. The Emperor and his mandarins were clothed in long silk garments, emblazoned with dragons and they sat cross-legged. Food was served on numbers of little tables, with many saucers and bowls; they ate with their fingers or used the ivory sticks provided. There was music, dancing, and performances by jugglers, tumblers, and acrobats which astonished Bell by their originality and expertise. Similarly, in the streets, he watched strolling-players and various sorts of entertainment. One man had trained a mouse to perform a dance, and then climb up and down a vertical chain four feet long, passing in and out of each link 'without missing a single one'.

The people were of medium height, slightly built, all with black hair and eyes. He saw no beggars but many soldiers; no one was allowed to carry arms in the city unless he was on duty. The garrison comprised 120 000. Bell took four hours to trot on horseback around the city walls. He saw few women, but was actually invited to choose a wife or daughter belonging to a Chinese gentleman with whom he had struck up a friendship. 'Ladies of pleasure' had their own well-ordered apartments in the suburbs, with a sign displaying their 'beauties, qualities and price'. They were not permitted on the streets.

During the centuries of the Ming Dynasty, Catholic missionaries from Portugal and Spain had established themselves at several Chinese ports, but the Manchus disliked them although the Emperor himself was tolerant and well-disposed to the Jesuits and Dominicans. They brought learning and skills; an observatory was built and Bell met the Jesuit in charge and examined the mathematical and navigational instruments there. It was a favourite place of the Emperor, and the Russians had brought four ivory telescopes constructed by Peter the Great himself. Clock-work time-pieces were also new to the Chinese. While Bell was there an Italian cardinal arrived from the Vatican, having travelled to Macao and Canton, and overland to Peking. He had come to examine a dispute which had arisen between Jesuits and Dominicans, about allowing Chinese Christian converts to continue certain traditional rites at the graves of their ancestors. Bell thought that the way the Emperor let them get on with it undisturbed, 'an instance of uncommon condescension'. With the death of the old Emperor a few years later, Christians began to fare less well.

European merchants had not succeeded as well as the missionaries in penetrating China. The object of the Russian mission was to establish trading centres and routes in China; furs could be exchanged for tea and silk. But the Chinese were suspicious and despite their outward hospitality, little was achieved by the Russians. Peking shops were full of small gold and silver bars; they only had one small brass coin. The bars were sold by weight and used as currency. When they wished to buy anything 'they cut off a piece of silver and weigh it, which is done in a trice'.

Bell visited several porcelain factories, intrigued by the mysteries of China-clay (kaolin) and the processes involved in the mixing of clay and granite, and the firing, glazing, and painting of their ware. They made no secret of their methods but Bell said he understood little and 'returned as ignorant as I went thither'. He was told that much of the ancient art had been lost and forgotten. Yet he was surprised to discover that the making of glass was unknown to them; when they first saw some prisms and pyramids of glass brought by the Jesuits, they thought they were just pieces of natural crystal. The Emperor promptly built a glass factory, which Bell was shown. Not lacking the essential materials for glass making, Bell thought that perhaps the Chinese ovens produced insufficient heat.

Printing had been used for centuries; 'they printed with stamps in the manner that cards are made in Europe'. We know now that the first printed book was made in China in the ninth century, and that movable type was developed there in the eleventh. Chinese paper, he thought, was made from silk or cotton, and was a very ancient art. It spread to Persia, Arabia, and via the Moors in Spain, to Europe, from the eighth to the twelfth centuries. At a splendid Royal Fireworks Display, to celebrate the New Year, Bell was lost in admiration at the spectacle of soaring rockets and coloured crackers of various forms lighting up the sky. The combustion of saltpetre, sulphur, and charcoal in fireworks had been known there for two thousand years, but its use as gunpowder was only recent.

Like the Persians, Chinese physicians knew nothing of European medicine, and although they used cupping, heat, bathing, and oint- ments, 'they seldom let blood'. Herbal remedies were the mainstay of treatment, but Bell did not mention acupuncture or, surprisingly, opium. The root of the Gensing plant was highly esteemed, and it was gathered only by certain employees of the Emperor, but Bell had never found it of any use. The custom of infanticide was widespread among the poor, as there were so many wives. The streets were searched each morning for rejected newborn, and taken into care. The binding of the feet of newborn females was also nearly universal. Ladies were seldom seen in the streets except in sedan-chairs; they probably had difficulty in walking. Bell was told that the custom dated from the time a beautiful princess, born with bird-like feet, took to hiding them with bandages. But it is more likely to have been a way of restricting female mobility.

The Great Wall, he was told, had been built in the space of five years, six centuries ago (it probably dates from the second century BC). It extended for 1200* miles; 'every sixth man in China was employed'. Constructed of huge stone blocks and bricks, and filled with earth to form a roadway fifteen feet wide, it ranged over the hills and mountains, twenty feet high. Fortified with square towers every hundred yards or so, it had proved a forbidding obstacle to invaders for many centuries. China itself, Bell thought, was already enclosed and sealed off by the ocean, the mountains and the desert and he doubted whether any nation, except perhaps the Russians, could contemplate invasion.

At a Royal Hunt, in an enclosed area of field and forest, ten miles from the city, Bell saw thousands of tents and men, lined up before the Emperor's pavilion. With bow and arrow, greyhounds and falcon, and fowling-pieces, they pursued deer, fowl, wild boar, and, as a climax on the final day, three tigers. Extending for mile after mile, surrounded by a high wall, they followed the Emperor on his palanquin, through his estate. 'It was a most delightful place'.

Return to St. Petersburg

The outward journey having taken them sixteen months and having spent four months in Peking, the Russians were anxious to make better speed on the homeward route; in fact it took them ten months. Bell himself said that at the appropriate time of the year he thought he could arrange to complete the double journey in six months. They crossed the Gobi desert on horseback in nineteen days, with changes of horse two or three times each day, and leaving the baggage wagons to trail behind. Leaving Peking on 1 March, they forded the river Tola on 3 April and reached the Selenga river camp at the Russio–Chinese border on 8 April. From there they travelled on the ice to Lake Baikal, which they were able to sail across, dodging the floes, and arriving at Irkutsk where they remained until 2 July, when all their baggage had arrived and they were again ready to resume their journey. Sailing up the Angara, they had to negotiate cataracts at three places, and their old enemies the mosquitoes renewed their torment. By 24 July they had reached Yeniseyk, and after a week's rest, they rode on horseback to the nearby river Kei, on which they spent some tiresome weeks floating down through a flat desolate countryside, to the river Ob. Entering it, the

* Now commonly estimated to be 1500 miles.

passage was swifter and they reached the town of Surgut on 11 September, there, turning down into the Irtysh on the 19th. With fresh winds and new crews they made Tobolsk by 2 October. During their stay there, they heard of the end of the twenty-year war between Russia and Sweden. There was much celebration.

The rest of the journey to Moscow was by sleigh and horseback— through the Aral Mountains, to Molotov on the Kana river, and then by-passing Kazan and making straight for Gorky through the forests east of the Volga. They reached Gorky in time to celebrate Christmas there and were back in Moscow on 5 January 1722.

III. MOSCOW TO DERBENT WITH THE RUSSIAN ARMY

Now that Sweden had surrendered her Baltic provinces and Peter I had secured for his country an ice-free seabord, he wished to show his people in Moscow that it was the creation of the Fleet which had brought his twenty-year struggle to its successful conclusion. When Bell returned from Peking in January 1722 he found that the Russian Court was in Moscow and great celebrations were in progress. In February, to demonstrate his naval strength to a people 'who had a strong aversion to shipping and maritime affairs', Peter arranged a spectacular naval cavalcade. Armed galleys, frigates, decorated barges, pilot boats, and smaller vessels by the score, were towed by teams of horses on huge sledges, through the streets of Moscow.

But soon, the Czar's thoughts were turning to the south and east again. The embassy to Isfahan had revealed the fragile, decaying state of the Persian Empire, and reports were now reaching him of threatening invasion of the Caspian lands, by Caucasians, Turks, and Afghans. The vital trade routes along the western shore of the Caspian were in danger. A great fleet and army was assembled below Moscow and in May they set sail down the Volga. Bell, invited to join the staff of the Emperor's chief physician, said that there were 15 000 soldiers and 300 ships in the armada. At Saratov, they were joined by 5000 Kalmucks, and when they reached Astrakhan, on 4 July, there were thousands of Cossacks assembled.

The Emperor and Empress sailed with the foot-soldiers in their fleet, while the horsemen marched along the shore route, and they joined up again in a bay of the peninsula of Agrakhansk, some two hundred miles to the south. A fort was built and Bell estimated that by the middle of August the army of 30 000 was ready to march. It was a hot and dusty route, lacking in water, and on one dreadful night 500 horses died from eating some poisonous shrub; Bell suspected the Roman wormwood or mugwort. There were over 300 wagons, each drawn by two oxen. From the mountains on their right they were harrassed by bands of armed men bent on stealing cattle. Periodic forays were necessary to protect their flank. The Empress and her ladies travelled in carriages.

On the approach to Derbent, on the Persian border, they were relieved to see approaching them, on 30 August, the Governor of Derbent, with his retinue of officers and magistrates, carrying the gold keys of the city on a cushion of brocade. The city formally surrendered, a Russian garrison was established, and Peter and his army marched through its streets, and formed their camp in vineyards to the south of the city. But disaster followed. A convoy of supply ships from Astrakhan arrived a few days later only to be dashed to pieces in a violent storm, with loss of most of its provisions. Their next goal was the port of Baku, one hundred and fifty miles south, there Bell would have seen more of 'that bituminous liquid called naphtha' which formed pools among the rocks near Derbent and which the Persians burned in their lamps. But there was no question of Baku surrendering; the Russians would have had to give battle. Peter I realized he was now in no position to do this, so he cut his losses, and leaving a garrison at Derbent, headed north. After an exhausting march of eleven days they reached their fort at Agrakhansk, 'having seen no rain since our landing on this coast'.

The Russian ships conveyed them eventually to Astrakhan where they were glad to arrive on 14 October. Here, although Bell does not mention it, the Emperor became ill with urinary infection and was not able to leave for a further six weeks. Meanwhile, Bell and a few others returned by boat to Stalingrad, and then travelled overland to Moscow, by a route he does not actually describe, where they arrived on 25 November. The Emperor and his wife arrived a few weeks later.

IV. LENINGRAD TO ISTANBUL

Bell's fourth journey, in 1737, was to Constantinople. Russia and Germany had been at war with Turkey since 1734. At the Sublime Porte there were ambassadors from Great Britain, France, and Holland, and Bell was requested to take certain proposals to the Ottoman Court, by the British ambassador in St. Petersburg and the Chancellor of Russia. He left on 6 December 1737 'with only one servant' who spoke Turkish. Winter travel by sleigh was a speedy affair; he was in Moscow by the 9th and mentioned the devastation consequent on the fire of the preceding summer. He reached Kaluga on the 12th, Sievsk on the 15th, and Kiev

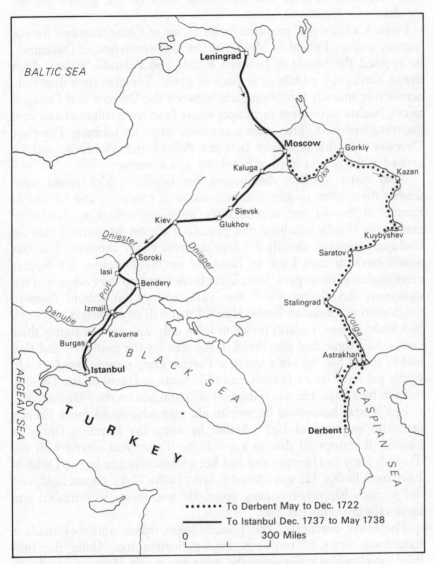

BALTIC SEA

Leningrad

Moscow

Gorkiy

Kaluga

Kazan

Oka

Sievsk

Kiev

Kuybyshev

Glukhov

Dniester

Saratov

Soroki

Iasi

Dnieper

Bendery

Prut

Stalingrad

Izmail

Volga

Danube

Kavarna

Astrakhan

Burgas

BLACK SEA

Istanbul

CASPIAN SEA

AEGEAN SEA

T U R K E Y

Derbent

•••••• To Derbent May to Dec. 1722

———— To Istanbul Dec. 1737 to May 1738

0   300 Miles

JOHN BELL IN RUSSIA: THIRD AND FOURTH JOURNEYS

on December 18th. Strangely enough, on the last few days, he had to ride horseback as there was insufficient snow on the ground for the sleighs.

From Kiev, he was provided by an escort of Cossack troops for the journey acrosss Poland to Moldavia. On the twenty-first of December, he crossed the boundary between Russia and Poland—'a deep ditch drawn across the middle of a spacious plain'. For nine days they rode across this sparsely inhabited plain between the Dnieper and Dniester rivers. Nights were spent in villages where Jews were common and kept the travellers' inns. They were a common target for robbers. The river Dniester was the boundary between Poland and Moldavia, and he arrived at the border town of Soroki on 30 December.

Now under Turkish domination, the Christian Moldavians were unable themselves to give him permission to continue, and he had to remain at Soroki for several days while authorities at Iasi were consulted. Finally reaching this provincial capital he learned that he could not continue directly to Constantinople by the shortest route, but would have to turn back to Bendery, on the Dniester, for further examination of his papers. Journeying there he noted the evidence of the customary devastation which the Turks always left behind them in neighbouring Christian lands. He said that half of Moldavia had been laid waste; it was Turkish policy to leave only sufficient to supply their garrisons. Plague had also raged in the area for the past year, and Bell had to spend five days in a hut in a Turkish camp outside Bendery. He finally got away on 12 January and rode south to Izmail on the Danube delta in four days. He was reminded of Astrakhan on the Volga delta.

In a Tartar household he met an old man who could speak French and who enquired of Bell whether he knew the Lorraine family in France. It transpired that as a youth the Tartar had served with the Turkish army in Hungary and had been taken prisoner by the Duke of Lorraine's forces. He was invited to serve in the Duke's household, and did so, very happily, for many years. He was always well treated and eventually given his freedom.

The lower reaches of the Danube were frozen and they made a hazardous series of crossings among floating ice. Along the hills bordering the Black Sea shore the going was rough. Here, said Bell, 'we are in the Ancient Kingdom of Thrace, now reduced to a Turkish province known by the name of Bulgaria'. There were ruins of old castles, and Greek monasteries. They reached Kavarna on 24 January, Burgas on the 25th, and Constantinople on the 29th of January.

Bell lodged with the British ambassador at Pera, during his

two-month stay there, carrying out his instructions, which he chose not to discuss. From a distance, he wrote, the city presented an attractive appearance, with its minarets and domes, its striking position on the Bosphorus, and the bustling shipping in the Golden Horn. But he found it noisy, dirty, congested (population 40 000), with myriads of narrow mean streets 'and a great number of nasty dogs'. Plague and other pestilential fevers were ever threatening; 'the Turkish authorities suffer all ships to enter port, without requiring bills of health at any time'. In the streets it was common practice to cross to the other side to avoid contact with anyone you suspected of 'distemper'. He added, 'Most people endeavour to get to windward of each other'.

He visited most of the famous sights but assumed that they were so well known that he said little about them. He rode out to inspect the viaducts, he went into the underground water cisterns, he visited the mosques and hippodrome, admired the Egyptian obelisk and the triple serpent column (from Delphi) and also the gardens which sloped down from the seraglio to the sea—'though it was not even safe to look at them with a spy-glass'. One morning he saw the Sultan on horseback, 'looking of a humane and peaceable disposition'.

When the army of the Grand Vizier set off for war in Hungary the ceremonial parade to the encampment outside the city lasted four days. The troops were accompanied by the various trades and artisans, in their distinctive clothes and badges, with banners and music. 'This raga-muffin crew made frightful figures, being naked to the waist, with sabres run through the fleshy parts of the arms, and besmeared with blood—a shocking spectacle'. On such an occasion Mohamed's standard—a horse's tail—was carried in procession and when war was declared it was hung at the gate of the seraglio.

Bell left the city on 8 April, carrying some dispatches to the Grand Vizier's Camp, then at Edirne, a town near the present Turko–Bulgarian border. He delivered them on the 13th and left for home on the 17th, by much the same route as he had come south. He arrived in St. Petersburg on 17 May 1738.

*

Bell retired to Antermony House in the parish of Campsie, Stirlingshire, in 1746 and died there thirty four years later. He had some fine tales to tell. Of Campsie, it was said, in 1845

If those times and places which are the best to read of are the worst to live in, the inhabitants of this parish must be held to have been fortunate beyond the ordinary lot of mankind, there being almost no events connected with it which can be called historical; and the names of its past or present inhabitants, that are most known, or are likely to be long remembered without its bounds, are those of Dr Bell of Antermony, the traveller; Mr Charles Mackintosh, the inventor of the celebrated waterproof cloth, which bears his name; and Mr James Bell, the celebrated geographer.

BIBLIOGRAPHY

Chambers, Robert. *A biographical dictionary of eminent Scotsmen*, 4 vols; I, p. 196 (1835).
The New Statistical Account of Scotland, 1845, Vol. 8, p. 244. Blackwood.
Peter the Great, Oudard, Georges. Trans. F. M. Atkinson. T. Werner Laurie, London (no date).
Peter the Great; his life and work, Massie, Robert K., Gollancz, London (1979).
Palmyra of the North; the first days of St. Petersburg, Marsden, Christopher. Faber & Faber, London (1942).

4

Alexander Hamilton in Colonial America
1744

DR ALEXANDER HAMILTON (1712–56) was one of the seven sons of
William Hamilton, professor of Divinity and principal of the University
of Edinburgh. He studied medicine there and obtained the degree of
MD in 1737. There is no definite evidence that he studied in Leyden
although he refers to the city and to Boerhaave (1668–1738) in his
journal. Emigrating to America in 1739, he settled in Annapolis,
Maryland, where an elder brother, John, was already established as a
churchman or physician. He made his journey to Maine in the summer
of 1744, after a period of ill health and fear of consumption. He kept a
journal and for some reason or other he gave the manuscript to an
Italian friend, in November of that year. It turned up, in the early years
of the present century, in a London bookseller's, and was purchased by
an American collector, William K. Bixby. It consisted of 278 pages of
neat handwritten script and was privately published in 1907, introduced
and edited by Albert Bushnell Hart, Professor of History in Harvard
University. It was subsequently issued by the University of North
Carolina Press, with an introduction and annotations by Carl
Bridenbaugh, in 1948. In 1971 it was reprinted by the Arno Press of
New York.

Professor Hart said that there were few contemporary descriptions of
the Colonies in America between 1730 and 1745, and he thought that
The Itinerary 'must henceforth be reckoned with as one of the best
sources of authority on the social life of the period'. With the assistance
of two graduate students of history Hart was able to construct a map of
Hamilton's journey, which was followed by one of them, and to identify
names and places. I have redrawn it, with a few minor omissions.

Hamilton married in 1747 and died in 1756, one year before the birth
of that celebrated American statesman of the same name. Doctor
Hamilton was thus a bachelor of thirty-three when he set off on
horseback with his negro servant Dromo, through the middle colonies

and New England colonies, along the Atlantic seaboard. There is no hint that he had previously travelled northwards and we soon appreciate that his eyes were fresh and observant. He was clearly a likeable young man with a warm personality, full of fun, disliking pomposity, intolerance, and religious bigotry, and not at all like the traditional portrait one may have in mind of an offspring of a Scottish presbytery of the eighteenth century. On most pages the reader will find something amusing or interesting, and, unlike many travel writers of that era, conversational encounters enliven the pages. The journey took four months, and they were on the road for nearly half that time, spending seven days in Philadelphia, eight in New York, and nine in Boston, on the outward stage—and five, ten, and eleven further days respectively in those towns, on the return trip. I thought it best to more or less combine his accounts of them, in separate sections.

OFF TO PHILADELPHIA IN THE MORNING

Hamilton and Dromo began their journey at eleven-o-clock in the morning of 30 May 1744. He had planned to cross Chesapeake Bay to visit friends at Newtown but 'contrary winds and bad weather' prevented this so they set off on the long road along the west shore of Delaware Bay and the Pennsylvanian bank of the Delaware River towards Philadelphia—a distance of some 120 miles, making an excursion southwards from the top of the bay, to Newtown. Many rivers, some of them small, others wide, flowed into the bay and river, so there were a number of ferries to cross—Patapsco ferry, Elk ferry, Bohemia ferry, Sassafras ferry, Cristin ferry, and the Skuylkill ferry at Philadelphia.

'The journey', he said, 'was only intended for health and recreation' so there was ample time for leisurely gossip and discussion. Indeed, along the road, and in the taverns, inns, and ferries, not to mention the many private homes he visited *en route*, there were to appear in the pages of his journal, a seemingly endless roll of characters to instruct, divert, and entertain him. His passage through the countryside at times recalls those tales of Chaucer and Borrow. He must have had a winning way with him and a good sense of fun. There was no lack of company wherever he found himself.

On that first day they went 26 miles, staying the night at the home of an aquaintance, enjoying 'a country dinner' with punch. The wife of his host was deaf 'so we were blessed indeed by a silent woman' and able to converse 'like a couple of virtuosos'.

On the ferry the next day, a captain of a tobacco boat decided to accompany him as far as the village of Baltimore. Hamilton was lectured on the therapeutic value of the Gensing plant which could be found thereabouts. He looked for it at one ferry 'as I had a curiosity to see a thing which has become so famous', but found none. Arriving at one inn they saw a drunken group 'riding off helter skelter as if the devil had possesssed them—each—like a bunch of rags tied upon the saddle'. The landlord was 'a fat, pursy man and had large bubbies like a woman'. They supped on fried chickens and bacon and were entertained by a demonstration of tooth extraction. The itinerant dentist practised on a housemaid—'a dirty piece of lumber'—using 'a great clumsy pair of blacksmith's forceps'. After 'much screaming and squalling' he pulled out something which 'resembled a horsenail more than a tooth'.

Next morning after 'a breakfast of dirty chocolate', they took of at six-thirty and at the Susquehanna ferry, which was a mile wide, they found the ferryman and his wife 'at their vittles'. This was 'a homely dish of fish . . . in a dirty, deep, wooden dish which they evacuated with their hands, cramming down skins, scales and all'. An argumentative passenger by the name of Thomas Quiet, 'a religious bigot . . . told me flatly I was damned without redemption'. Hamilton informed him that his name was inappropriate. At the Elk ferry, the young ferryman 'plied his tongue much faster than his oar' in telling them that for the local English folk 'he had the honour to stand pimp in their amours'. At the Bohemia ferry, he slept in the same bedroom as the landlord, his wife and daughters. At Newtown, he met his friend Dr Anderson and dined with him. In the yard of a local tavern they were amused by the way the female baboon showed her indifference to anyone of the female sex—'especially the black'.

Newcastle, he said, had been founded by the Dutch. It had a courthouse and a church. He stayed at the Indian King Tavern where he was joined by three Pennsylvanians who assured him that their State was superior to Maryland— better pasture and more civilised. One of them, a clownish, rough-spun character, went to great lengths trying to pass for a gentleman. 'Damn me, gentlemen, excuse me', he would say, 'I am a plain honest fellow; all is right-down plain-dealing with me', by God . . . '. At an inn below Wilmington, as they neared Brandywine River, 'There was a dish of swearing and loud talking . . . and . . . after dinner we fell upon politicks and the expected French war'. They deliberated on the meaning of the words 'declaration' and 'proclamation', concluding that the former was for war and the latter for peace. At times Hamilton had to hide his mirth behind a handkerchief—'I slurd a laugh with nose-blowing as people sometimes do a fart with coughing'.

Chester was a pretty, neat village, with a bridge over the Delaware half

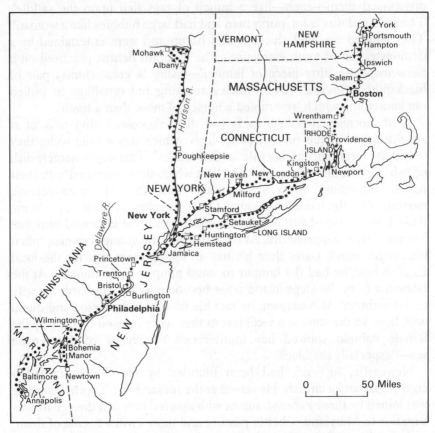

ALEXANDER HAMILTON IN COLONIAL AMERICA, 1744

a mile below it, which put him in mind of Chelsea, near London. The common type of salutation on the road was 'How d'ye' or 'How is't'. At Darby, in the last inn before Philadelphia, there was a fine long argument between a Quaker and a boatswain about 'the lawfulness of using arms against an enemy'. 'The Quaker thee'd and thou'd it through his nose to perfection'—and the bosun swore.

PHILADELPHIA

Hamilton stabled his horses at The Sign of the Three Tons in Chestnut Street and obtained lodging nearby. The local countryside was 'level and pleasant . . . fruitful in grain and fruits, pretty well watered and abounding in woods'. Bread, flour, and pork were the principal staples. There was a fine prospect of the Delaware, in which a ship, a sloop, and a schooner were visible, with the coast of New Jersey on the other side. The streets were not paved and the majority of the houses were 'mean and low'; they were made of brick and some had balconies. The town was laid out 'in rectangular squares . . . uniform . . . but destitute of variety'. There were no steeples but there were a few good buildings— The State House (Town Hall), The Assembly House (Independence Hall, later), and a couple of churches. He thought it resembled 'an English country market town'. On two days each week, in Market Street, there was the 'largest market in America'. It was very hot and 'awnings of painted cloth or duck' hung over many of the doors and windows of the shops. At dusk buckets of water were thrown over the pavements which provided 'a sensible cool'. The local water was excellent, and there was a pump 'every fifty paces distant'.

Philadelphians were a business-like people and shopkeepers opened up at 5 a.m.. In general, they were inquisitive of strangers, but not very friendly. They did not like 'Maryland folk'. Little attention was paid to strangers unless they were 'of more than ordinary rank . . . or came for trade'. 'A Pennsylvanian will tell a lie with a sanctified, solemn face; a Marylander, perhaps, will convey his fib in a volley of oaths'. There was no scarcity of 'men of learning or good sense' but ladies seldom appeared in the streets, and never at public assemblies 'except at churches or meetings'.

There were two large meeting houses for the Quakers—'an obstinate, stiff-necked generation and a perpetual plague to the governors'. They were influential in Assembly. It was a sombre place—'I was never in a place so populous where the gout [taste] for public, gay diversions prevailed so little'. Some Virginians had recently tried to arrange a ball—'but the ladies were not interested'. There was no dancing or music—'their chief employ, indeed, is traffic and mercantile business which turns their thoughts from these levitys'.

Hamilton spent a week in town, meeting the citizens, the Governor Thomas, and some doctors, one of whom showed 'some good anatomical preparations of the muscles and blood vessels injected with wax'. One day in a tavern

There were Scots, English, Dutch, Germans and Irish; there were Roman catholics, churchmen, presbyterians, quakers, Newlightmen, methodist, seventh day men, anabaptists, and one Jew. The whole company consisted of twenty-five planted around an oblong table in a great hall stoked with flys. The company divided into committees in conversation; the prevailing topic was politics and conjectures of a French war. A knot of Quakers there talked only about selling of flowers and the low price it bore . . . .

He 'enjoyed entertaining conversation' at the Governor's Club, which met every night at the tavern; the Governor attended once a week. One night the topic was 'the English Poet's'; they also discussed Cervantes. But politics, religion and trade were the main topics. He heard about the debates and conflicts in the Legislature where 'the ambition and avarice of a few men' were usually at work.

One day, outside his lodging, he watched a boxing match between a master and his servant'.

The master was an unwieldy, pot-gutted fellow, the servant muscular raw-boned and tall; therefore though he was his servant in station of life, yet he would have been his master in single combat, had not the bystanders assisted the master and help him up as often as the fellow threw him down. The servant, by his dialect, was a Scotsman; the names he gave his master were no better than little bastard, and shitten elf, terms ill applied to such a pursy load of flesh.

News of war with France arrived during his stay. The proclamation from the King of England was read from the Court House steps. Some four thousand people collected, 'two hundred gentlemen attending Governor Thomas' and there was a long procession, with 'thirty flags and ensigns from the harbour . . . a parcel of roaring sailors . . . eight or ten drums' all producing 'a confounded martial noise'. The fitting out of privateers was planned, and Governor Thomas said 'This province shall not be lost by any neglect or oversight of mine'.

ON TO NEW YORK

From Philadelphia to New York, about eighty miles as the crow flies, their ride took Hamilton and Dromo through Bristol, Trenton, Princeton, Kingston, Brunswick, Perth Amboy, then across the waters to

Staten Island and Coney Island, and on to the York ferry from Long Island to Manhattan. They were on the road for three days, crossing several ferries and dining, or staying at inns with such names as The Sign of the Wheat Sheaf, The Sign of the Black Lion, The Sign of Admiral Vernon, and The Sign of the King's Arms.

At Trenton they met a Dr 'Cadwaller' (almost certainly Thomas Cadwalader (1708–79) of Philadelphia, a well known Quaker physician, pioneer of inoculation, founder of the Philadelphia library and the first to teach anatomy there by dissection. He left a classic account of lead colic and lead palsy, entitled '*An essay on the West Indian gripes*' (later shown by Benjamin Franklin to be due to the consumption of Jamaican rum which had been distilled through lead pipes). Cadwalader enquired about things in Maryland, 'its politicks and legislature', and whether Hamilton knew a Dr Hamilton of Annapolis. He had heard that he was ill and likely to die. Hamilton replying 'Here he is'. So they got on to the subject of religion, agreeing that there was much nonsense in ceremonies and that religion should wear a 'genuine simple and plain dress'.

Princeton, in New Jersey, was a small village, without a college. The first buildings went up ten years later and its name—the College of New Jersey—so remained until 1896. The aim of the founders was to provide an institution in the Middle Colonies, like Harvard and Yale in New England, and William and Mary in Virginia.

In an inn at Kingston, after a dish of tea served up by a pretty, smiling girl, a wagon drew up in which were two Irishmen, a Scot and a Jew. Over their drinks there was a long dispute about the Old Testament— the day of creation, Moses, and the Jewish sabbath. Of the day of creation, the Scot enquired, 'Had that evening no morning then?'. They were joined by 'an old don on horseback'. In rustic dress, he talked of mathematics and physics and astrology. The landlord told Hamilton that the old philosopher was a well known local character who 'understood mathematics to a hair's breadth' and who had actually written to Holland enquiring about the longitude there.

With a Dr Farquhar at Brunswick he enjoyed some pickled oysters, and on the ferry there, met a boy jockey. At the Inn in Perth Amboy, there was an old bachelor at breakfast, who he was told, lived alone, fed his own poultry, milked his own cows, and dressed his own vittles— without help or servant—although he owned most of the houses in the town. Staten Island reminded Hamilton of the Scottish highlands in parts, with its large pastures and great stones. He thought that the island was about eighteen miles by six or seven. He tasted his first dish of clams here, but was surprised by the manner of saying grace—'solemn face, head down, holding up hands for half a minute'. He had difficulty coping with an over hastily-stuffed mouth of rye-bread, butter, and fried clams. It was a long dinner and the clams took some chewing; they began to get cool, so the landlady called for a bedpan, 'which she used by way of a chafing dish to warm our clams'. Hamilton's sleeve got caught on the handle of the pan and knocked it over. 'The landlady was a little ruffled and muttered a scrape of Dutch.'

From Coney Island to the York ferry, some seven miles, past orchards of cherry trees and many stone fences, they had twenty-four gates to open. Dromo, failing to understand the dialect of a negro girl of whom he had enquired the way, told Hamilton that she was 'a damned black bitch'. On the ferry there was a beautiful wife with her husband. She had fine features and complexion, black eyes and hair, and an elegant shape. 'She had an amorous look, and her eyes, methought, spoke a language which is universally understood . . . her voice had music in it.'

NEW YORK

The Dutch, explained Hamilton, were the first settlers here, and the city (Lower Manhattan) 'makes a fine appearance for above a mile all along the river'. The best streets ran parallel to the water, the wooden wharfs had stone foundations, and there was much shipping about. It looked 'a very rich place'. He took lodgings in Broad Street and looked around. Although the Dutch language and customs were declining, the majority of the houses were 'after the Dutch model with their gable ends fronting the street'. A few were built of stone, some of wood, but most were of brick—'many covered with pan tile and glazed tile, with the year of God when built, figured out with plates of iron on the front'.

In the streets, water was sold from huge casks carried on sledges; the water came from neighbouring springs and was hard and brackish. There were many handsome women in the streets, walking, or carried in light chairs. Their umbrellas were often painted or adorned with feathers. Women of fashion promenaded in the evening. He learned that although 'the government is under English law', many of the important positions in the Assembly were held by Dutchmen. There was a mayor, a recorder, aldermen, and a common council. The Town House stood on Broad Street, and the Exchange, with its wooden pier, was at the waterside.

The day following his arrival was a Sunday so he went to church, a building of about a hundred feet long and eighty wide, with 'a heavy clumsy steeple of freestone, fronting the street called Broadway'. The congregation was 'above a thousand', the singing was good and the Minister discoursed well on the Christian virtues. The church gallery was supported by 'wooden pillars of the Ionic order with carved work of foliage and cherub's heads, gilt betwixt the capitals'. There was also two Dutch churches and one synagogue.

Down at the fort and battery, there was the Lieutenant-Governor's house, a chapel, fine gardens and a terraced walk. On a semicircular bluff rampart there were handsome brass guns. He was told that here, of an evening, a stranger could 'fit himself with a courtesan, for it was the general rendezvous of the fair sex of that profession after sunset'. There was 'a good choice of pretty lasses among them, both Dutch and English', but he decided he was not 'so abandoned as to go among them' and went off to supper at Todd's Tavern.

Todd was an old Scot, full of 'quaint saws and jack-pudding speeches', and there was a lot of heavy drinking among the characters who met there. Each night, the Hungarian Club met, and there was much talk. Another old Scot, sheriff of the city, had 'a homely, carbuncle kind of countenance with a hideous knob of a nose which he screwed into a hundred different forms while he spoke'. He met several doctors there—a surgeon from the fort, another from a man-o-war who only drank water, and 'a grave old don with a yellow wig and greasy gloves'. He met the son of surgeon David Knox of Edinburgh 'in whose shop I had learnt pharmacy'. 'We talked over old stories.' There was a Major Spratt, tall, thin with a dry cough and 'phthisical'; he was 'half seas over in liquor'.

There were many toasts, to King or some Governor usually, and they were called 'bumpers'; there were too many, he found, for him. Meals were long and noisy. At one there was bacon, chicken, and veal. At another, veal and beefsteaks. Green peas were also usually served. On one occasion, a doctor asked that peas be omitted from his plate, but the negro maid forgot, and when the doctor saw the peas 'he began to stare and change colour . . . I thought he would be convulsed, but he started up and ran out of doors' and did not return. We might wonder whether this was something more than a simple aversion—a reflexly induced syncope or epilepsy, perhaps.

On one evening there was 'a tolerable concerto of music performed by one violin and two German flutes'. On another a young gentleman from Boston sang 'in an extraordinary voice', accompanying himself with a violin. 'The whole company were amazed that any person but a woman or a eunuch could have such a pipe and began to question his virility; but he swore that if the company pleased he would show a couple of as good witnesses as any man might wear.' He went on to imitate a dog, a cat, a horse, a cow, and 'the cackling of poultry' to perfection.

Hamilton played backgammon, and watched chess, read the newspapers, wrote letters and visited the two coffee houses in the city. The Post went off once a week—to the north and south. But talking and walking and dining were his main recorded activities. Dodging the 'bumpers' was essential if one wished to wake up with a clear head. At one tavern a discussion arose about a poem which had been published in a newspaper. At one time, a lawyer gave a disquisition on 'nominatives and verbs'. There was a necessity, he said, that there should be a verb to each nominative, 'in order to make sense'. Hamilton got into an argument with one doctor about the effect of the moon on fluids in general. The New York doctor talked much about 'attraction, condensation, gravitation and rarification; he told us he was troubled with open piles and with that, from his breeches, pulled out a linen handkerchief all stained with blood and showed the company'. Hamilton asked him if the moon affected his piles in the way it did menstruation. But the doctor thought that the moon had nothing to do with 'our distempers'. And so the week passed.

UP THE HUDSON RIVER TO ALBANY

A week or so after arriving in New York on his northward journey, Hamilton boarded an Albany Sloop carring some eight other passengers, and sailed up the Hudson River. On the first day they collected a cask of spring water from an old 'Scots-Irishman tenant farmer' on Nutting Island (Governor's Island). There were no nuts but plenty of myrtle berries, juniper and ipecacuanha plants; hay and barley had been damaged by worm. Greenwich, a little town of eight or ten houses, lay on their starboard side and a few miles on, there were cliffs which rose near a hundred feet on the New Jersey shore—the Palisades. They passed places with odd names—Dunder Barrak (Dunderberg), a mountain on the east bank opposite Peekskill, in the district called the 'Highlands'. St. Antony's Nose was a rocky promontory on the east bank, near Bear Mountain. Cook's Island, a mere 'rock ten paces long and five broad', was so named because a certain cook from a man-o-war was buried there; it was a wild and solitary place, the water ninety fathoms deep, so that a large sloop could sail close upon the shore, its boom brushing leaves from the overhanging branches of trees. This was the 'Narrows of the Highlands'. There was Deoper's Island, Butter

Mountain, and Murder Creek (scene of a massacre by Indians), and Dancing Hall where 'sixty or seventy years ago some young people from Albany, making merry and dancing, were killed by some Indians who lay in ambush in the woods'.

At Poughkeepsie, where they arrived on the fourth day, a garrulous and tiresome Dutchman and his wife, left the sloop. He talked a strange mixture of Dutch and English—'a confusion of language'—contributed to, Hamilton thought, by his endless preoccupation with the Tower of Babel, its height, shape, and construction, as revealed by many pictures of it he had studied. He also advised Hamilton how to manage his constitution, when, for a while, he rested from 'his constant and darling theme'. Drinking and whoring, he said, made you thin and sickly; six weeks of abstinence and 'your belly and cheeks would be like mine'. On learning that Hamilton was a doctor, he told him 'Your art is vain. Find me a doctor among the best of you that can mend a man's body half so well as a joiner can help a crazy table or stool.'

Hamilton and Dromo were the only passengers who could speak no Dutch. One Englishman, a Minister, was fluent in Latin, Greek, French, and Dutch—but he also was bothersome. He read to them from a book about the microscope and said that he had studied under Boerhaave in Leyden. He also bragged about his 'mathematicks' but Hamilton suspected 'he knew not the difference between a cone and a pyramid, a cylinder and a prism'. A lecture on the microscope, it seemed, was 'tiresome to one who had seen Leeuwenhoek and some of the best hands upon the subject'—another bit of tarradiddle as Hamilton was only eleven years of age when Leeuwenhoek died in 1723. The Dutchman and the Minister discussed the meaning of the word 'superstition' and the book of Ecclesiasticus—to the amusement of the crew and passengers.

From another Englishman, living with his wife and seven 'wild and rustic' children, in a log cabin about forty miles from New York, they bought a pail of milk. Although obviously very poor, the cabin was clean and neat, and they possessed some finery, a dozen pewter spoons, a framed mirror, a set of tea dishes, and a musket. The Minister thought that wooden plates and spoons would have been good enough, and the water in that wooden pail might have served as a mirror. If they sold their finery, he said, they could have purchased some wool and made yarn. The children, 'who stared like sheep at my laced hat and sword', picked some blackberries for the visitors.

In a tavern at Poughkeepsie, a small village on the right bank, set in high woody land, the Minister and Hamilton met a Justice of the Peace 'who seemed to have the greatest half or all the learning of the county on his face, but as soon as he spoke, we found that he was no more learned than other men'. With him was a tailor, a member of a Moravian sect who shared everything communally and taught that religion had been corrupted by the laws. 'The tailor's phizz was screwed up to a sanctified pitch, and he seemed to be under a great sorrow for his sins or else a "hatching some mischief in his heart".'

About half way to Albany was Esopus Island, and near the Catskill mountains the river was some two miles wide. On the fourth day of sailing, as they approached Albany, they encountered a rumour that a search party of Canadian Indians was near, hunting a French couple with a price on their heads. The man was said to have been a priest, and the female, his lady. He was wanted by the Governor in Canada, 'dead or alive'; if dead his scalp was to be taken and also 'the consecrated flesh from his thumb and forefinger'. Others said that the two were French spies. Perhaps it was 'all a plausible fiction'.

ALBANY

Albany, about one hundred and sixty miles from New York, lay on a rising hill on the west bank of the Hudson, twelve miles below its junction with the Mohawk River at Cohoes Falls. There was a square stone fort, manned by three hundred English soldiers, with a bastion at each corner, each with eight or ten guns, most of them thirty-two pounders. Within the fort were two brick houses. The majority of the town's population of four thousand were Dutch. There were three main streets, one running up from the fort, and two parallel with the river. The town itself was surrounded by a ten-foot high palisade, made from the trunks of pine trees a foot thick. There was a block house every two hundred feet and five or six town gates.

There were three markethouses, an English church, a Dutch church, and a Town House, the two latter with spires. The Dutch were hard working and thrifty, 'owning more land than cash', and engaged in the wampum trade—making black and white beads from clam and conch shells (from the West Indies), drilling and stringing them, for sale to the Indians. They also sent good hay and grain down the river in their twenty-four sloops. Dutch houses were clean and neat, with wooden floors scrubbed smooth and fine, spacious rooms, and beds so hidden in their alcoves that one could walk through the large house without seeing a bed. Kitchens were hung with 'earthen or Delft plates all around the walls', but they lived frugally and in the winter seemed to subsist chiefly on salt provisions. With their morning's tea they would have 'raw hung beef sliced down in chips in the manner of parmesan cheese'. At one supper 'we smelt something very strong like burnt oatmeal which they told me was an animal called a skunk, the urine of which could be smelt at a great distance . . . '.

Old ladies in their head-dresses, large pendants, and short petticoats, looked quite comical; 'they stare upon one like witches'. Young men called their sweethearts 'luffees . . . and a young fellow of eighteen is reckoned a simpleton if he has not yet a luffee'. The Minister formerly lived in Albany and conducted Hamilton around the town. 'We went into twenty or thirty houses where I went through the farce of kissing the women, a manner of salutation which is expected from strangers . . . this might pass for a penance, for the generality of the women here, both young and old, are remarkable ugly.' Hamilton was sorry for the young men who had seen no other girls.

From Albany he visited the Cohoes Falls—eighty feet high and nine hundred broad—where the noise drowned out human voices, and where, in Spring, when the ice broke up, it sounded like the guns at Albany. Schenectady was a nearby Indian trading village on the Mohawk River, with a few brick houses set in a plain surrounded by thick pine woods. Back in Albany, he dined with the Fort surgeon and learned that the town school accommodated some two hundred children, and that most of the doctors were Dutch—'empirics all, having no knowledge or learning but what they acquired by bare experience'. Herbal remedies were the standby. At a tavern dinner he met the town worthies; the viands and wine were good, the conversation rude and clamorous. One sunny afternoon Hamilton dozed off against a wall, and wakened to find that a cow had taken a handkerchief he had put over his head. 'I pursued her for some time before I recovered it, when I suppose the snuff in it made her disgorge, but it was prettily pinked all over in holes.'

A Captain Blood, a 'downright old soldier', at the Fort, said he was a nephew of the notorious Captain Blood who had tried to steal the crown jewels in the Tower of London in 1671. Another captain said he had been at the siege of the Flemish town of Namur in 1695, when King William III, took it from the French. 'Scots Willie', another old soldier, recalled seeing Lord Dundee fall at the battle of Killecrankie in Scotland, in 1689. Dundee led the Jacobite army against the Royalists.

But by 2 July 'I now began to be quite tired of this place where there was no variety or choice, either of company or conversation'. The Dutch language was rough sounding and the people, although civil and hospitable, were 'rustic and unpolished'. They were very retiring, 'their whole thoughts being turned to profits'. So down the Hudson he went, calling at various places for water and provisions. They failed to get any milk at Buttermilk Island, where the river was a mile broad and its banks vertical. An old man named Williams was there, with three sons and a daughter, struggling to make a living by providing fish and cutting timber to be sent down river. Hamilton wondered how they survived in winter. At one place they bought a bucket of milk and three fat fowls for ninepence. It was owned by a Dutchman who had eighteen children, nine boys and nine girls; the girl of sixteen being 'handsome'. By 6 July he was back at New York where he found his horses 'in good plight' and made arrangements to leave on the next stage of his journey in a few days time.

NEW YORK TO BOSTON

Their route was along the north shore of Long Island, across The Sound to New London, Connecticut, and then up through Rhode Island into Massachusetts. Leaving New York on the tenth of July they arrived in Boston on the eighteenth. Two traders, Parker and Laughton, accompanied them some of the way. They caught the ferry to Long Island at 7 a.m. and breakfasted at The Sign of the Sun in Jamaica, at 10 a.m., on 'bread, mouldy cheese, stale beer and sour cider'. At Hempstead, 'a very scattered town standing upon the great plain to which it gave its name', they lunched at The Sign of Guy of Earwick. Parker was mightily taken by a pretty girl and 'would fain have stayed the night'. She had 'fevers' which Parker thought he could cure 'if she would submit to his directions'. But they finally persuaded him to mount his horse. The road was long, smooth, but indistinct, through flat grasslands, with winding brooks and small oak bushes. Losing one's way was easy; they saw few people, and they were surprised to see how they ran away 'as fast as bucks upon the mountains'. One boy, lurking in a bush, dashed away in a frightened manner, when approached. They spent their first night at Huntington, at The Sign of the Half Moon and Heart. (It was at East Hampton, Long Island, that Dr George Huntington saw those families with an hereditary disease of the brain which he described in 1872. His father and grandfather had practised medicine there. The tainted families with Huntington's chorea sailed from Suffolk to New England in 1630. One wonders whether the furtiveness of the folk Hamilton saw that day, was perhaps a symptom of mental disorder.)

In the Huntington inn there was a 'band of the town politicians', one of whom, 'with a worsted cap and great black fists' was the local quack.

A cobbler by trade, he had gained some repute when he cured an old woman of 'a pestilent mortal disease', so decided to 'lay aside his awls and leathers and fell to cobbling human bodies.' There were also three buxom girls to whom Parker made strenuous courtship. Their names were Phoebe, Lucretia, and Betty. Phoebe was an Indian, but Betty was 'the top beauty of the three'.

They were on the road at 6.30 a.m. next day, breakfasted at The Sign of the Bacchus, and reaching a ford at 10 a.m. from where they could see the coast of New England across The Sound. At Brookhaven they met a fellow 'who showed us several antick tricks, such as jumping half a foot high on his bum without touching the floor with any other part of his body. Then he turned and did the same with his belly.' He also stood upright on his head. He told them he was seventy-five and 'swore damn his old shoes if any man in America could do the like.' The travellers, in turn, regaled him with some tall stories, Hamilton explaining that he came from 'Calliphurnia.' 'The old chap was mightily elevated at this and damned his old shoes twenty times over.'

That evening, they lost their way and were tormented by 'muscettoes' and went to bed supperless at Brewsters. When he woke in the morning, Hamilton found in his room 'two great hulking fellows with long black beards', in one bed, and another 'a raw-boned boy.' They left earlier, and a loom in the corner suggested they may have been weavers.

At Southold, there were windmills, and they stayed the night at a Mrs More's in 'a company of patched coats and tattered jackets' to the sounds of 'Damne ye, Jack' and 'Here's to ye, Tom'. A pedlar and a Dr Hull compared their respective professions. All went to their beds in the same chamber. In the King's Inn, at their next stop at Oyster Pond, on 13 July, there were some handsome country girls to attract Parker, 'who was apt to take flame upon all occasions'. For lunch they had fat pork and green pease, and then boarded the ferryboat which took them across eighteen miles of water in some three-and-a-half hours. New London was a desolate sort of place along the waterside. Gunfire at sea had been heard, and there were more speculations about the French.

At Stonnington, next day, a landlady described as 'an enormous heap of fat' had daughters and maids with names such as Thankful, Charity, Patience, Comfort, and Hope. 15 July was a Sunday—a pagan term that was forbidden—and they discovered that one could not travel on the Sabbath. Neither could you whistle or sing, for the landlord scolded Parker for so doing. Hamilton sought refuge in a book. For supper there was only bread and milk.

They were relieved to catch the Narragansett ferry next day, which took them to Newport, Rhode Island, where the countryside was like 'an entire garden of farms' and 'remarkable for pretty women as Albany is for ugly ones'. Hamilton met a Dr Moffat there, an Edinburgh graduate, 'an old acquaintance and school friend of mine'. He also met a Dr Keith and a Dr Brett and he was taken to see some paintings by 'one Feykes . . . a most extraordinary genius'. 'Keith passed for a man of great gallantry here!' He possessed 'a cabinet of curiosities' which sported such items as torn fans, fragments of gloves, whims, snuff boxes, girdles, apron strings, laced shoes, shoe heels, pin cushions, hussifs, and 'a deal of other such trumpery'. Hamilton observed that Keith was 'visited by very airy and frolicsome ladies of the town'.

He spent the night at Moffat's and was provided with some letters of introduction to 'the fraternity at Boston.' At Bristol, next day, he met a Boston barrister named Lightfoot, an Oxford graduate, who had dispensed with a wig. He wore a straw hat when the weather was hot and said that country folk suspected he was some sort of spy. There was a rumour of a French attack on Nova Scotia. They journeyed on together, and at Dedham, their last stop before Boston, Lightfoot 'was obliged to vent a deal of billingsgate and swear a string of lusty oaths' before he could retrieve a lemon which the landlady's daughter had 'secreted'.

BOSTON

Boston was then the largest city of America and Hamilton said its population was between twenty and thirty thousand; it was actually about sixteen thousand. He found it more rewarding than Philadelphia and New York and stayed for nine days on his northward journey, and another eleven when he was returning south. He lodged with a French lady near Beacon Hill and from the garden of the house he said there was a fine view of the town and the two-mile long peninsula on which it was built. Charleston lay across the water, about a hundred ships lay in the bay, and on one of the islands was a fort. Twelve miles out at sea was a lighthouse, the first in America. It was a flourishing commercial centre—ship building, fishing, farming, lumber, and general merchandise.

The lower chamber of the Town House (State House), a long one with a row of wooden pillars down the middle, was called 'The Change'. There were many large warehouses and a new market house built by Mr Faneuil, near the waterside. The present-day Faneuil Hall is of a later date. Hamilton posted some letters at The Change, where he saw some French officers arranging the exchange of prisoners of war. 'They were very loquacious after the manner of their nation . . . their discourse interlaced with oaths and smut.'

At the Sun Tavern he met a variety of people. The Physical Club and the Scots Quarterly Society met there; Hamilton gave a donation to the latter. Its president was a Doctor Douglas—a well-known physician who had been educated in Edinburgh and Leyden. He had founded the Medical Society of Boston in 1736. Hamilton found him domineering and argumentative—'a compleat snarler' who talked slightingly of Boerhaave, calling him 'a mere helluo librorum, an indefatigable compiler who dealt more in books than observation'.

At a book sale, Hamilton bought a copy of Homer's Iliad. The auctioneer was a witty, taunting young fellow who explained that in his collection 'there was everything concerning popes, cardinals, antichrist and the devil'. Nearby he saw a parade of Indian Chiefs. 'The fellows had laced hats, matchcoats and ruffled shirts'; they had been deputed to explain to the 'Eastern Indians' that the English were their friends, and the French their enemies. He observed that already the Indian Nation seemed to have been divided into two on the basis of religion—Catholic and Protestant. There was a Colonel Wendal with the Indians and Bridenbough has pointed out that he was a Dutch ancestor of Dr Oliver Wendell Holmes. At church, Hamilton heard a sermon which was really 'a lecture in philosophy'—all about such things as the specific gravity of air and water, the expansion and condensation of clouds, distillation and the chemistry of nature. The preacher was 'a conceited prig with superficial knowledge and ostentatious words'.

On the road to Cambridge, to see Harvard College, with an acquaintance, they passed some 'French Mohawks'—an old man on horseback, and a young one with his squaw on the saddle behind him. The men were dressed 'a la mode François, with laced hats, full-trimmed coats and riffled shirts'. On their two small roan horses they were travelling some seven hundred miles to the west. In Cambridge there were 'pretty country houses'; the college building was 'square-shaped', with a handsome clock and a good bell, and a large courtyard. They met the President and saw the library of three or four thousand books.

Another visit was to the Fort in the bay where a good view of the lighthouse was obtained through a spyglass. There was a central courtyard, a water well, a flagstaff; sentries paraded on the ramparts, where there were many guns. It was a commanding defensive position.

The city folk were hospitable and he paid many visits. There were fewer Quakers as they had been 'banished from the first settlement' because they were troublesome. So there was music and dancing available, and the town 'abounded in pretty women'. There were plenty of 'educated folk' too. In the taverns there was good food and talk, but less drinking than in New York. New gun batteries were being constructed and privateers were being fitted out. There was talk of a proposed attack on the French at Cape Breton as Bostonians feared for their fishing grounds. Hamilton ate salt cod dressed with egg and butter sauce, there was plenty of beef and puddings. In several conversations he detected 'a vein of that subtilty and acuteness so peculiar to New England genius'. But there was also a lot of 'High Court maxims and silly doctrines'. A local clergyman caused much gossiping. He had lost his living 'for being too sweet upon his landlady's daughter, a great belly being the consequence'. He met a Captain Patty, six feet tall, with a humped back—'the tallest hump I ever saw'. There was a little dapper fellow named Clackenbridge, 'disputatious and semi-learned'; he was a woman-hater and 'decried marriage as a political institution destructive of human liberty'. The president of one club in a waterside tavern, was a 'pot-bellied doctor'. In a second meeting with Dr Douglas, Hamilton had to listen to a condemnation of a new German book on surgery.

A Scottish lady he used to visit, had 'a great round red face' and two 'vivacious and shapely daughters'. One was coquettish and wore 'a robe de chambre of cherry-coloured silk, laced with silver round the sleeves and skirts, and neither hoop nor stay'. Alas, both girls had 'vile squints' so that their eyes looked 'two ways'. The mother suggested that she could help Hamilton to set up in medical practice in the city; she was rich.

In another house there was 'a great mixture of girls', one being small and lively—'a proper mixture of the French mercury and English phlegm'. Dining one day with a Mr Arbuthnot, Hamilton complimented his daughter on her playing of the spinet. The father 'asked me if I could pay her no other compliment but that, which dashed me a little'. One day, in a street, a Boston girl, on hearing that he was a Maryland physician, exclaimed 'O Jesus, a physician, deuce take such odd looking physicians'.

On one visit he was amused with the behaviour of 'a white monkey from the Mosquito shore'. The monkey was exceedingly fond of his mistress—'bussing her and handling her bubbies like an old rake. One might envy the brute, for the lady was very handsome'. The monkey 'laughed and grinned like a Christian'. All this lead Hamilton to deliver himself of a few lines of evolutionary thought.

The progress of Nature is surprising in many such instances. She seems by one connected gradation to pass from one species of creature to another without any visible gap, interval, or discontinuum in her works; but an infinity of her operations are yet unknown to us.

He described a diversion known as 'hawling the fox'. It took place outside the town at a pond 'about a quarter of a mile across'. A rope was laid across it and a fox was tethered to a tree stump near the end of the rope, on one side. Hidden in nearby bushes were two strong chaps and it was they, not the fox, who held the rope. On the other side a passer-by would be challenged to try and pull the fox across the water by tugging on the rope; a reward was promised. A simple fellow agreed to try and allowed the rope to be tied around his waist. He then started to tug but found himself being quickly hauled across the pond 'while the water hissed and foamed on each side of him as he ploughed the surface'. The fellow, 'a poor pill-garlick', could not believe a fox could have such strength. It recalls the old custom of tug-of-war across a village pond.

A young Frenchman with the name La Moinnerie also lodged in the same house as Hamilton. He was a law graduate of Paris who had come to Boston after trying for a time to start a practice in Jamaica, only to be caught up by the war. He feared he might be taken prisoner and not allowed to return to France. He was a gay, companiable young man, adept at cooking, and for ever explaining to the maid how things should be prepared. They became good friends—taking lessons from each other in their respective languages. At first they had to talk in Latin. When leaving Boston after his second visit, Hamilton wrote that

Nothing I regretted so much was parting with La Moinnerie, the most lively and merry companion I had ever met with, always gay and cheerful, now dancing and then singing though every day in danger of being made a prisoner.

Hamilton commented on how the Frenchman differed from an Englishman. The latter, 'upon the least misfortune are for the most part clogged and overclouded with melancholy and vapours.' When Hamilton finally left Boston, La Moinnerie was sad and 'kept fast hold of my stirrup for about a quarter of an hour'.

BOSTON TO MAINE

The road took them along the coast of Massachusetts, on 28 July, through Charleston, Lynn, Marblehead, Salem, and Ipswich, and on to New Hampshire, with its short coast line of about fifteen miles, and across the water at Portsmouth, into Maine.

At the fishing town of Marblehead, population of about 5000, the main occupation was catching and drying the cod. 'The land was covered with fish scales' for some 200 acres around the town, and there were ninety fishing sloops in the harbour. A minister played a violin and a flute at The Sign of the Dragon. At Salem 'a pretty place being the first settled in the northeast', he put up at the Ship Tavern. A conversation with a Justice of the Peace ran on to 'the enthusiasm now prevalent in these parts and the strange madness that had possessed some people at Ipswich, occasioned by one Woodberry' an itinerant preacher who 'pretended to inspiration'.

The owner of a fine house and estate he visited in Salem, also had 'a strange taste for theological discussion'. 'Original Sin', thought Hamilton, 'was no more than the monstrous and deformed offspring of theological heads' and he hoped he would only hear of it when he took 'a cathartic of emetic in order to promote the operation if it proved too sluggish'. Curiously, he made no reference to the notorious witch trials of 1692.

Near Ipswich he noted that the houses were 'thick planted', which reminds one that today, a not uncommon roadsign in rural New Hampshire, is one that just says 'Thickly Settled'. 'An inquisitive rustic' accompanied him as far as Portsmouth and Hamilton recorded a sample of their 'dialogue' as 'a specimen of the many of the same tenor' he had had on his journey. It ran thus:

Pray Sir, if I may be so bold, where are you going? Prithee, friend says I, where are you going? Why, I go along the road here a little way. So do I, friend, replied I. But may I presume, Sir, whence do you come? And whence do you come, friend says I. Pardon me, from Singleton's Farm, replied he, with a bag of oats. And I come from Maryland, says I, with a portmanteau and baggage. Maryland, said my companion, where the devil is that there place? I have never heard of it. But pray sir, may I be so free as to ask you your name? And may I be so bold as to ask yours, friend? Mine is Jerry Jacobs at your service, replied he. I told him my name was Bombast Huynhym van Helmot, at his service. A strange name indeed; belike you are a Dutchman, Sir—a captain of a ship, belike? No friend, says I, I am a High German alchemist. Bless us, you don't say so; that's a trade I never heard of; what may you deal in, Sir? I sell air, said I. Air, said he, damn it, a strange commodity. I'd thank you for some wholesome air to cure my fevers which have held me these two months.

Hamilton arrived at Portsmouth on 1 August, met Governor Wentworth of New Hampshire, and learned that the town's population was about five thousand. He visited a fort on Newcastle Island, which had 30 guns, and a garrison of 60 men, whose small arms, he thought looked a bit rusty. He had dinner in the guard room and was told that they kept geese to help guard against a surprise attack,as at 'the Roman Capitol'. New Hampshire was a rocky, woodland of a State, divided into townships, and not shires or counties as elsewhere. Their chief trade was in ship masts and fishing. His trip by ferry across to Maine, and a nine-mile ride to the village of York, completed his journey to the North. He seems not to have had any reason for visiting York, he said next to nothing about it, and one suspects, as he returned to Portsmouth the same day, that it was only undertaken so that he could truthfully say he had travelled from Maryland to Maine and back.

FROM MAINE TO MARYLAND

They went by the same route back to Boston, where they arrived on 4 August and stayed until the 17th, renewing acquaintances and making new ones. Then, on through Rhode Island to New London, but instead of recrossing the Sound, they continued along the Connecticut coast to New Rochelle and on to the ferry across the East River to York Island (New York), where they arrived on the 31st.

He continued to record the people he met, noting their dress, foibles, and prejudices. At Wrentham, in Massachusetts, there was a tall thin physician 'with a weather-beaten wig, an old striped collimancoe banian* and an antique brass spur upon his right ankle, and a pair of thick-soled shoes tied with points'. He could be heard in his bedroom at his long, loud and earnest prayers, pleading for 'fullness of grace and the blessings of regeneration and the new birth'. His words, said Hamilton, 'abounded in tautologies' and were accompanied by much groaning of spirit.

At an inn in Providence, Rhode Island, there was 'a rabble of controversy between two learned Divines' in a room whose walls were covered with illuminated texts about such things as the Golden Rules, The Wise Men of Gotham, The King and the Cobbler, and the Cannons to batter the Tower of Babel.

At Newport he spent a few days with Dr Moffat and used his microscope to examine a spider, the eye of a fly, the wing of a moth, and some small feathers. Here, there was less religion, the people were outspoken and frank. They railed against English taxes so that 'collectors and naval officers . . . dare not exercise their office for fear of the fury and unruliness of the people'. There was much talking and

* A 'banian' is a loose jacket of flannel; 'collimancoe' has eluded me but sounds Scottish

planning about ship-building and privateering, while at the Philosophical Club, there was discourses on all sorts of topics. One evening it was
all about Bonny Prince Charlie, Lord Lovat, and General Wade. At
other times 'We tossed the news about.' And, of course, there was the
inevitable comical fellow, one who, on this occasion imagined 'he could
discover longitude with an instrument made of whale bone and cartilage
or gristle'. He also thought that although Sir Isaac Newtown and Lord
Veralum (Sir Francis Bacon) were great men, unlike him, they were not
immortal. He had the idea of 'cutting the American Isthmus in two so to
make a short passage to the South Seas . . . and how to make a machine
with little expense by the help of which ships may be dragged over that
narrow neck of land with all the ease imaginable, it being a trifle of one
hundred miles . . . '. Sometimes, however, Hamilton found the
discourses 'stupid and fanatic' and of 'no benefit to mankind or public'
and went off to bed. But Rhode Island remained in his mind as 'the most
delightful spot of ground I have seen in America'.

He crossed the mouth of the Connecticut River, by ferry and toll
bridge, and at Guildford an old man showed him a stone bridge over a
brook, which was made of 'one entire stone about ten feet long, six
broad, and eight or ten inches thick, being naturally bent in the form of
an arch, without the help of a chisel to cut it into shape'. At Newhaven,
the College, (Yale), consisted of a three-storied wooden building about
two hundred feet long, in the centre of the town. In the middle of the
building was 'a little cupola with a clock upon it'. The college was the
gift 'of a private gentleman of the place' but it was not so pleasing as
Harvard, and had fewer students. Hamilton went on by way of Milford,
Stratford, Fairfield and Norwalk, to Stamford, his last stop in
Connecticut. At Norwalk a man with a cancer of the lip asked for advice;
'I told him that the only treatment is to cut it out'. When Dromo
'grinned like a crocodile and showed his teeth hideously', some
frightened children asked if he was coming to eat with them. Leaving
Connecticut at Horse Neck, Hamilton mused that the state had 'ragged
money, rough boards, and enthusiastic people but could raise 6000 men
able to bear arms'.

Back in York Island (Manhattan), there were stark-naked Indians
gathering oysters; some sort of feast was being prepared; 'an entire ox
was roasting on a wooden spit' and everybody, including the crew of a
man-o-war were 'getting drunk as fast as they could'.

He stayed in New York for ten days, leaving on the 11th of
September, sorry to leave his friends but anxious about too much drink.
He took the same road back to Philadelphia and was there in three days.

After another six days, he set off for home, reflecting that he had got a better impression of the Quaker city on his second visit. It was a politer place than New York, there was less drinking, and the citizens were good at business. But it seemed to be 'an accomplishment peculiar to all our American colonies'.

On the second day out, poor Dromo 'tumbled down, horse, baggage and all' but no harm was done. At Wilmington he saw a carter whom he thought must have been an hermaphrodite. 'All above, from the crown of his head to the girdle seemed masculine, the creature having a great, hideous, unshorn black beard and strong coarse features, a slouch hat, cloth jackets, and great brawny fists; but below the girdle there was nothing to be seen but petticoats, a white apron, and the exact shape of a woman with relation to broad round buttocks . . . I thought it most prudent to pass by peacably.'

He dined with his friends at the Manor House in Bohemia and on the following day was asked to see a doctor's wife suffering from 'hysteric palpitations', or 'as they call it—a wolf in her heart'. On the 24th a man asked him if he had heard about 'The War'. It seemed that 'The Queen of Sheba, or some other such Queen, had sent great assistance to the King of England . . . if that was true . . . they would certainly kill all French and Spaniards by next Christmas'. Hamilton noticed the faces of the people were pale and washed out; there had been a lot of fever during the summer.

He was home on September the twenty-seventh, estimating that he had travelled some 1624 miles.

In these my northern travels I compassed my design in obtaining a better state of health . . . I found but little difference in the manners and character of the people in the different provinces I passed 'thro, but as to constitutions, complexions, air and government, I found some variety . . . [they were] . . . better and happier in the north . . . [where there was] . . . better air . . . and . . . the people of more gigantic size and make.

*

Hamilton remained in Annapolis for the remainder of his days and was elected to the Lower House of the Maryland Assembly in 1753, three years before his death at the age of forty-four. He wrote a pamphlet on the prevention of small pox and was a founder member of 'The Ancient and Honourable Tuesday Club', a dining club with eight original members, 'designed for humour, and . . . a sort of farcical Drama of Mock Majesty', of which, as 'Loquacious Scribble Esq.', he was the historiographer. The manuscript records of the club, with caricatures from his pen, are in the care of the Maryland Historical Society. Perhaps the reader will not be surprised to learn that after this merry soul departed—the club never met again.

BIBLIOGRAPHY

Hamilton's Itinerarium, being a narrative of a journey etc, in 1744, by Doctor Alexander Hamilton. Edited by Albert Bushnell Hart. LL D. Privately printed by William K. Bixby, St. Louis, Missouri (1907).

Gentleman's Progress: the Itinerarium of Dr Alexander Hamilton, 1744. Edited with an introduction by Carl Bridenbaugh. University of North Carolina Press, Chapel Hill (1948).

Hamilton's Itinerarium. Arno Press Reprint, New York (1971).

5

Tobias Smollett's Travels through France and Italy
1763–1765

IN June 1763 Dr Tobias Smollett, MD of Chelsea, London, took the road to Dover on his way to the south of France, where, he hoped 'the mildness of the climate would prove favourable to the weak state of my lungs'. But if his lungs were weak, his passions were still strong and he was soon raising his dander about 'the worst road in England'. The modern traveller might still agree with him, however, that 'the avenue to London by way of Kent street . . . is a most disgraceful entrance' and that 'a foreigner, in passing through this beggarly and ruinous suburb' must still wonder if he will ever see Westminster.

Smollett was then forty-two years of age. He was born in Dalquhurno, a farm on the banks of the Leven, near the village of Renton in Dunbartonshire. He attended the local grammar school and went to Glasgow University, and for a few years he was apprenticed to a surgeon in that city. At the age of twenty he set off for London, and in 1742 he gained a warrant from the Navy Board as a surgeon's mate. His experience in the Royal Navy formed the basis of his first novel, *The adventures of Roderick Random*, published in 1848, and which Hazlitt considered his best. When Roderick, a young surgeon apprentice, was examined by the Navy Board, he was castigated for being a Scot ('we have scarce any other countrymen to examine here') and for having served only three years apprenticeship; in England he would have had to serve seven. After being questioned about trepanning, one of the examiners enquired what he would do if 'a man should be brought to you with his head shot off?'. Roderick confessed that he had not seen any method of cure proposed in any of the systems of surgery he had studied. There were smiles and some further questions, followed by a rumpus among the examiners about the treatment of abdominal wounds, which served to terminate Roderick's interrogation.

Smollett served for two years in the West Indies, and in *Roderick*

Random and in his *Account of the expedition against Carthagena*, there are vivid descriptions of life at sea, the crowded quarters of the lower decks, the hardships, discipline, wretched food, and the terrible fate of the sick and wounded. Hornblower again.

He returned to London and in 1744 we find him with a wife from Jamaica, in medical practice in fashionable Downing Street (where the young Boswell later found lodgings). He does not seem to have stayed there long and from 1750 he lived in Monmouth House, Chelsea. By this time he had obtained the degree of MD from Mareschal College, Aberdeen, on payment of a fee and the likely recommendations of such London-Scottish sponsors as Smellie, Armstrong, Douglas, and the Hunters—all medical friends of his.

He was not successful in medical practice and by 1752, when he published his only medical paper—*An Essay on the external use of water*—he had more or less taken up a literary career. He had written medical reviews and edited Smellie's *Midwifery* but most of his energy was increasingly devoted to editing, translating, and writing—pamphlets, articles in magazines and books on political, historical, social, and literary topics—and novels. *Roderick Random* had brought him fame at the age of twenty-seven, *Peregrine Pickle* followed in 1751, and *Humphry Clinker* in 1771, the year he died. He worked hard for many years and although he must have been able to earn a satisfactory living (one of the first English novelists to do so), he was generous and extravagant. Monmouth House was a place where of a Sunday evening there were good things to be enjoyed by his 'unfortunate brothers of the quill . . . beef-pudding and potatoes, port, punch and Calvert's entire butt-beer'. There were distinguished visitors such as John Hunter, Wilkes, Garrick, Sterne, Goldsmith, and that 'great CHAM of literature', as Smollett called Dr Samuel Johnson.*

Overcritical and quarrelsome, he had to spend three months in the King's Bench prison in 1759, convicted of libelling an admiral in one of his articles. In 1762 we find him asking for a loan of money from John Hunter.

THE TRAVELS

Overworked, dogged by money-troubles and ill-health, grief stricken at the death of his only child, a girl of fifteen, Smollett and his wife set off in the company of two ladies he had promised to chaperone, attended by his trusty servant 'who had lived with me for a dozen years, and now

---

* CHAM, explained Boswell, was the title of the Sovereign of Tartary, 'which is well applied to Johnson, the Monarch of Literature'.

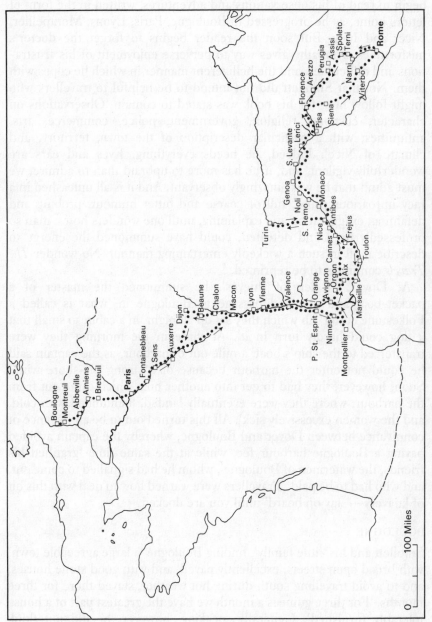

TOBIAS SMOLLETT IN FRANCE AND ITALY, 1763–5

refused to leave me'. His readers, we can be sure, wish him well as they begin to read of his observations and adventures, written in the form of letters home, as he progressed to Boulogne, Paris, Lyons, Montpellier, Nice, and Italy. But soon the reader begins to forget the doctor's misfortunes; sympathy gives way to perverse enjoyment of his frustrations and difficulties, and the belligerent manner in which he copes with them. Not that Smollett did not intend to be helpful to travellers who might follow him, for his book was stated to contain 'Observations on character, customs, religion, government, police, commerce, arts, antiquities; with a particular description of the town, territory, and climate of Nice'. Indeed, he heeds everything. Eyes and ears are wonderfully vigilant, and, if he has more to upbraid than to admire, we must admit that he was amazingly observant. And it is all unleashed in a racy uproarious prose, full of coarse and bitter humour, probing and defaming, exaggerating and explaining, until one wonders how a man so professedly tired and defeated, could have summoned the energy to describe it all in such a wickedly entertaining manner. No wonder *The Travels* continues to be reprinted.

At Dover, 'a den of thieves', he summoned the master of a packet-boat and obtained passage to Boulogne in 'what is called a Folkestone cutter', in which they sat up all night 'in a cabin so small that a dog could hardly turn in it'. At three in the morning they were transferred to the ship's boat, a mile out of harbour, as the captain said he could not enter the harbour because of a strong off-shore wind. Soon, however, they had to get into another boat which came out from the harbour, where they were eventually landed, 'benumbed with cold, and the women excessively sick'. All this turned out to be an instance of connivance between Dover and Boulogne, whereby the captain avoided paying a Boulogne harbour fee, while at the same time 'gratified his friends, the watermen of Boulogne', whom he had signalled to come out, and who had to be paid. Travellers were warned how to deal with this bit of knavery—'stay on board' until you are docked.

BOULOGNE

Smollett and his 'little family', finding Boulogne 'a large agreeable town, with broad open streets, excellently paved' and with good stone houses, and to avoid travelling south during hot weather, stayed there for three months. 'For three guineas a month we have the greatest part of a house tolerably furnished'. Generally speaking, however, he did not think French homes as comfortable as English; the furniture was 'of clumsy workmanship', there were no feather beds or carpets, doors and windows seldom closed properly, but table-linen was plentiful and the cutlery good. Cleanliness was not a characteristic, there were smelly places, and some habits were quite indecent. He did not like to see a French lady 'who shifts her frowsy smock in presence of a male visitant, and talks to him of her *lavement*, her *médicine*, and her *bidet*!'. He knew of one lady 'handed to the house of office by her admirer, who stood at the door, and entertained her with *bon mots* all the time she was within'.

Although it was said to be 'one of the dearest places in France', he estimated 'that a man may keep house in Boulogne for about one half of what it will cost him in London'. There was an upper and a lower town, the former 'a kind of citadel' with a high wall and rampart, and a pleasant tree-lined walk with fine views. The *noblesse* lived there 'and never mix with the others'. In the larger, lower town, lived the *bourgeois*—and more conveniently. The harbour was shallow and there were two stone jetties. There were convents, churches, seminaries—and 'a hospital, or workhouse, which seems to be established upon a very good foundation . . . under the direction of the bishop'. There were several hundred inmates who worked 'according to their age and abilities'.

'The inhabitants of Boulogne may be divided into three classes; the noblesse or gentry, the burghers, and the canaille.' The gentry were 'vain, proud, poor, and slothful' who chose not to farm and live in their country houses, leaving their estates to decay. 'They have no education, no taste for reading . . . they hate walking,' and spent their time in dressing up 'and adorning their bodies'. They were 'helpless in themselves, and useless to the community'. The peasants 'often rendered desperate and savage, by the misery they suffer from the oppression and tyrany of their landlords' were a pitiful lot. Smollett did not live to see the inevitable Revolutionary storms.

'The bourgeois of this place seem to live at their ease.' There was a lively trade with England, including smuggling. The sea-faring community were a hardy, raw-boned type, who 'propagated like rabbits'. The fishermen went 'a great way out to sea, sometimes even as far as the coast of England'. There were many artisans, shopkeepers, and merchants. The bourgeois had 'soup and *bouilli* at noon, and a roast with a salad, for supper; and at all their meals there is a dessert of fruit'.

'The beef is neither fat nor firm . . . the veal is not so white, nor so well fed as the English veal; but it is more juicy and better tasted. The mutton and pork are very good.' There were fine poultry and hares and 'excellent soles, skates, flounders and whiting, and sometimes mackerel'. The oysters were large but 'coarse'. The Smolletts were well supplied with fruits of all kinds; strawberries, gooseberries, cherries, corinths, peaches, apricots, and pears. 'I have eaten more fruit this season, than I have done for several years.' The wine, to their disappointment, was 'very small and meagre'. 'The French inhabitants drink no good wine; nor is there any to be had', unless one dealt with one of the local British wine merchants who could provide some of the Bordeaux *en route* by sea to England.

Smollett enjoyed his summer there, making friends, talking to travellers, and listening and questioning them about all sorts of things. Anecdotes and vignettes are set down with relish. At one dinner party, where 'the best cook I ever knew' served up 'about twenty dishes', there was a gentleman at the head of the table 'tall, thin and weather-beaten, not unlike the picture of Don Quixote after he had lost his teeth'. A little sea captain, 'who had eaten himself black in the face, and with napkin under his chin', reminded Smollett of Sancho Panza 'in the suds, with the dishclout about his neck, when the Duke's scullions insisted upon shaving him'. (Smollett had translated Cervantes's book into English, some years previously.)

The religious houses and practices interested him. 'I know not whether I may be allowed to compare the Romish religion to comedy, and Calvinism to tragedy. The first amuses the senses, and excites ideas of mirth and good-humour; the other, like tragedy, deals in the passions of terror and pity.' English girls attended some of the convent schools 'where they learn scarce anything that is useful, but the French language; but they never fail to imbibe prejudices against the protestant religion . . .'. Of one seminary he wrote;

There was among the monks one Père Charles, a lusty friar, of whom the people tell strange stories. Some young women of the town were seen mounting over the wall, by a ladder of ropes, in the dusk of the evening; and there was an unusual crop of bastards that season. In short, Père Charles and his companions gave such scandal, that the whole fraternity was changed; and now the nest is occupied by another flight of these birds of passage. If one of our privateers had kidnapped a Capuchin during the war, and exhibited him, in his habit, as a show in London, he would have proved a good prize to the captors; for I know not a more uncouth and grotesque animal, than an old Capuchin in the habit of his order.

There were a few regulations, 'ordonnances', and laws to rail against. His books were confiscated on arrival, for inspection 'lest they should contain something prejudicial to the state, or to the religion of the country', but through the offices of an 'avocat' and the English ambassador in Paris, he recovered them from the director of the *douane* at Amiens. But a particular 'species of oppression', he learned, was the *droit d'aubaine*, whereby the effects of a foreigner who died in France, were seized by the King. Only the Swiss and the Scots were exempted.

During his stay, he continued to worry about his health and his prospects. The air was cold and moist, 'unhealthy'. An English military 'general', returning to retirement in England, after service with 'his Sardinian majesty', assured him that the climate of Nice was very suitable for those with 'disorders of the breast'. 'A gentleman of the faculty' returning from Nice also recommended it, while another, 'far gone in a consumption', had improved in Languedoc the previous winter. A local physician recommended cold baths and Smollett, though troubled by bouts of coughing, expectoration, and fever, decided there was no 'imposthume' in his lungs—so he 'plunged into the sea'. He caught a fresh cold, but persisted with the bathing and grew better. He talked much about the merits of cold and warm baths, referring to Hippocrates and Celsus, and various experiences of his friends and colleagues. He was certainly anxious and depressed at times, singularly naive about his theories. His last letter from Boulogne ended with 'It is a moot point whether I shall ever return. My health is very precarious.'

PARIS

Journeying to Paris by way of Montreuil, Abbeville, and Amiens, 'the landlords, hostesses and servants of the inns upon the road' did not 'receive you as in England' and you had to put up with 'the most mortifying indifference', although you knew they were 'laying schemes for fleecing you of your money'. At the gate of Paris the ladies had to stand in the street while the douane searched their coach. They stayed at a hotel in the Faubourg St. Germain and the doctor rented a carriage so that he could escort the ladies to 'the remarkable places in and about this capital'—the Luxembourg, the Palais Royal, the Tuileries, the Louvre, the Invalides, Trianon, and Versaille. Smollett knew Paris and was interested to see the new square laid out by Louis XV at the end of the Tuileries gardens, named after him, and with 'a good equestrian statue' of him in the centre. Later, it was to be 'Place de la Revolution', where his successor, Louis XVI met his fate, and still later, 'Place de la Concorde', with an Egyptian obelisk replacing the statue.

But everything seemed smaller than he remembered, a thing which puzzled him, and which he had previously experienced elsewhere. Versaille was 'a dismal habitation . . . the apartments are dark, ill-furnished, dirty and unprincely' and 'the collection of 'busts, statues and pictures' in Paris generally, did not impress him. At the Palais Royal he was 'bewildered in such a profusion'. He had seen the 'great magazine of painting three times' and found it too large to appreciate. I suppose many a young visitor since then, has been discouraged and exhausted in the art galleries of the Louvre, when an hour with the Impressionists in the nearby Jeu de Paume, would have served him better. The Trianon reminded Smollett of a pigeon house, but he admired the porcelain in the factory of St. Cloud, comparing it with that of Dresden and Chelsea. The streets of Paris were very narrow, and the houses high 'with a different family on every floor'. There was 'a scheme on foot for supplying every house with water, by leaden pipes, from the river Seine'.

But the greater part of his two letters from Paris, that October, dwells on its inhabitants. He lashed out. The shopkeepers and tradesmen were, of course, quite dishonest; they cheated. But it was the hotel valets who upset him most. They lay in wait for you; you have to hire them—they were difficult to shake off. They took over all your arrangements—'your tailor, barber, mantuamaker, milliner, perfumer, shoemaker, mercer, jeweller, hatter, *traiteur* [eating-house keeper] and wine-merchant'— and they profited well.

He wrote scornfully of the ladies and gentlemen of fashion. Of the ladies, he said, 'when I see one of these fine creatures sailing along, in her tawdry robes of silk and gauze, frilled, and flounced, and furbelowed, with her false locks, her false jewels, her paint, her patches, and perfumes; I cannot help looking upon her as the vilest piece of sophistication that art ever produced'. Girls were not educated but taught only 'to prattle, to dance and play at cards' before they made their debut in the *grande monde*. Then, their faces 'were primed and painted' in white and rouge, the former 'plastered' about the neck and shoulders, and the rouge 'daubed . . . from the chin up to the eyes, without the least art or dexterity'. 'Without this horrible masque no married lady is admitted at court, or in any polite assembly'. And just as their features were concealed under these 'ungracious colours . . . so their heads are covered with a vast load of hair, which is frizzled on the forehead' and completely whitened with powder. Every lady's head of hair had the same white colour 'from the moment she rises till night'.

As for the gentlemen, no Smollett reader will be surprised to learn that they were even 'more ridiculous and insignificant than the women . . . Of all the cox-combs on the face of the earth, a French *petit-maître* is the most impertinent'. The men, he acknowledged, were 'by no means deficient in natural capacity' but they also suffered from a 'preposterous' education. They learned how to pray in a Latin they did not understand, how to dance and fence, and how to pay compliments indiscriminately in a set of ridiculous phrases. Mingling with females from an early age, a young man becomes expert on their customs and humours. He attends at their toilette, 'and grows wonderfully alert in performing a thousand little offices'. He adjusts his lady's dress and hair, 'squires her everywhere' (which the doctor found agreeable), and seemed to dedicate his whole time to her, pluming himself on his gallantry. He would sooner part with his religion than his hair, 'the ornament upon which he bestows much time and pains'.

He knew of one man who suffered from headache and 'a defluxion on his eyes' who dismissed his physician on being advised to have his head 'close-shaved' and to bathe his eyes daily in cold water. He 'lost his eyesight and almost his senses, and is now led about with his hair in a bag, and a piece of green silk hanging like a screen before his face'.

France, said this happy traveller, was 'the general reservoir from which all the absurdities of false taste, luxury, and extravagance have overflowed the different kingdoms and states of Europe. The springs that fill this reservoir, are no other than vanity and ignorance'.

Perhaps, wishing to mollify the reader, he admitted that charges of insincerity and meanness, were not well-founded in the case of the French. He was also prepared to stress that when he talked of the French nation, he excepted 'a great number of individuals, from the general censure'. He respected the talents of many great Frenchmen who had distinguished themselves in the arts and sciences. As a race they had a vivacity and gay disposition one could envy—but 'they are the greatest egotists in the world'.

THE ROAD TO MONTPELLIER

Smollett's baggage had been dispatched by sea to Sète, 'the sea-port of Montpellier', from where he hoped to proceed to Nice by boat. He also wished to see the Roman antiquities at Nîmes and to test the 'boasted air of Montpellier', and, as we shall see, to consult the 'celebrated Professor F——, who is the Boerhaave of Montpellier'.

They decided to travel by post-chaise, by way of Dijon, to Lyon. The French custom was for the postmaster to find the horses and guides, and the traveller to hire a coach. They left Paris on October the thirteenth 'with six horses, two postillions, and my own servant on horseback'. There were fifty-nine posts to Lyon and they travelled about twenty miles a day. The highways were safe although they did not meet any of the *marrechaussée*—the mounted troopers who policed the highways—a service Smollett thought was needed in England. They usually breakfasted in an auberge at about ten-o-clock in the morning, ordering 'a poulard [a fattened pullet] or two to be roasted' and wrapped in a napkin, with bread, wine and water, for a picnic lunch in the coach during the afternoon. They had laid in 'a stock of tea, chocolate, cured neats' [ox] tongues, and *saucissons*, or Bologna sausages', so that, like many a modern traveller, the doctor 'found these transient refreshments much more agreable than any regular meal I ate upon the road'.

Fontainebleau reminded him of the New Forest in Hampshire although it was rockier and hillier, and more agreeable.The peasants looked poor, there were few enclosures and a great scarcity of cattle. They saw a man ploughing with a 'jackass, a lean cow, and a he-goat, yoked together'. He thought that 'husbandry in France will never be generally improved, until the farmer is free and independent'. They reached Macon on the fourth night, and at the gate of Lyon avoided a search with a tip. It was 'a populous and flourishing city . . . on the confluence of two large rivers'; the bridge over the Rhone looked too slight and its arches too small, to cope with the torrents which must sometimes descend on it. They rested there for a day, setting off in the morning in a fog so dense that they could not see the head of their foremost mule. In Lyon they had hired a berline (a four-wheeled covered carriage) drawn by three mules. The driver, Joseph, was 'a sober, sagacious, intelligent fellow' who knew the South well and who kept them amused with his anecdotes—but 'a knave' needless to say.

But they soon reached 'summer weather' along the banks of the Rhone 'through a most romantic country'. The road to Avignon ran straight but travellers to the south 'generally embark in the diligence at Lyon, and glide down this river with great velocity'. In good weather it was safe as far as Pont St. Esprit where the arches of the bridge were small and the boat might be upset in the turbulence. But passengers could get out and rejoin the boat below the bridge. Boats going up river were drawn by oxen 'which swim through one of the arches of the bridge, the driver sitting between the horns of the foremost beast'.

At one place there had been a robbery a few days before, so Smollett got his servant to load his 'musquetoon' with 'a charge of eight balls'. This 'blunderbuss' invariably attracted attention; it was called a *'petit canon'* and when it fired into the air the crowd would scamper off like a flock of sheep. They saw a naked body hanging from a gibbet and 'another lying broken on the wheel'.

They ate well, the Burgundy was satisfactory, but Smollett tired of the smell of garlic and the roasted thrushes served up in vine leaves, always half raw as the French liked them. The red partridges were twice the size of the English ones, and the hares were large and juicy. Milk was scarce; 'we were obliged to drink our tea without it'. There was almost routine grousing about the price of everything—hotel rooms, meals, hire of carriages and so on—and incessant squabbling, and bullying of servants. He regretted one noisy dispute, however, about a carriage at Sens, only, though, when he discovered that the man he had abused was the local *seigneur*. 'I was much mortified to find that I had treated a nobleman so scurvily.' He explained to the reader that the weather and his asthma had made him particularly peevish that day. In any case, the nobleman had been no better dressed than himself. We catch a glimpse here of the doctor in his 'grey mourning frock under a wide great coat, a bob-wig without powder, a very large lace hat, and a meagre, wrinkled discontented countenance'. He was a bit of a snob himself, despite his protests about the lack of 'antigallican spirit' of the English in Paris who all adopted the French style of dress there, and which he himself also appears to have done.

Entering the province of Languedoc, they breakfasted at Bagnole, 'a little paltry town', and, as they approached Nîmes, excited at the prospect of the Pont du Gard, their drivers put his mules to full gallop. Expecting to see it in some state of ruin, Smollett was delighted when he found it 'as fresh as the bridge at Westminster'. Raised by the Roman colony of Nîmes, it stood over the river Gardon, conveying water to the city. Admirably preserved, its three tiers of arches 'presents the eye with a piece of architecture, so unaffectedly elegant, so simple and majestic' which everyone could appreciate. He said it was 174 feet high and 723 feet long (modern guide books usually give figures of 166 and 900 feet) and explained that the water flowed along the top channel. A 'passage for foot travellers' had been made at the base of the second tier of arches (in the sixteenth century) and the 'citizens of Avignon' had added a road bridge alongside 'for horses and carriages of all kind' (in the eighteenth century). Modern visitors will know that this now hums with traffic between Nîmes and Uzes, but those golden, massive stones, some weighing as much as six tons, fitted together without mortar or cement, stand in eloquent tribute to the Roman engineers of nearly two thousand years ago.

So enchanted was he by the sight of this ancient monument that he said that if he lived nearby he would 'take pleasure in forming the parties to come hither, this summer, to dine under one of the arches of the Pont du Gard, on a cold collation'. Today he might enjoy the sight of campers and canoists, but in high summer he would have difficulty in finding a quiet spot under one of its arches. Sparks would soon be flying.

He was equally transported by the two other famous ruins in Nîmes—the amphitheatre and the Maison Carré (so-called because of its oblong shape). It was 'almost miraculous', and we can agree with him, that they were preserved; the amphitheatre probably escaped quarrying because the Visigoths converted it into a fortress. When Smollett was there the arena was 'filled up with houses' and some quarrying was going on. The Maison Carré had been a temple and was 'ravishingly beautiful . . . the whole world cannot parallel it . . . a man need not be a connoisseur in architecture' to appreciate the beauty of its pillars and columns, its frieze and cornice, and its general proportions. Now, it is a museum—a building which is said to have been in continuous occupation, by man and horse, for twenty centuries.

MONTPELLIER

Here, the people were sociable and good-tempered and had 'a spirit of commerce'. For the first time, he said, he encountered that 'gaiety and mirth' for which the French were so celebrated. The markets were excellent, but the wine was 'strong and harsh'; there were good liqueurs. There was a Protestant community; they chose to assemble privately in the country for their Sunday 'conventicles'. The weather was very hot at first, but soon it began to rain and blow; Smollett started to cough. There was fever, 'spitting and lowness of the spirits' so he consulted a resident English doctor, but does not say what came of it. He then made up his mind to seek the advice of Professor Fizès, 'the lanthorn of Medicine'. He had planned to see the University, the Medical School and the famous Botanical Garden, but he is silent about them. He did not meet Fizès, but conjured up a picture of him in which speech, appearance, and behaviour, were particularly unsavoury. From what he had heard, he said he had 'no desire to converse with him'.

Whatever his reason, and it may have been fear of being labelled a consumptive, the subsequent 'consultation' reveals a patient of pathetic sharpness, and a professor who was either very careless or unversed in Latin.

Smollett sent an account of his ill health to the professor by valet, enclosing a fee. It was written in Latin, presumably to impress.* He gave his age as thirty-four (he was forty-three); this was not a slip as he mentioned it again in his second letter. He described how, for some years he had been subject to bouts of fever, cough, expectoration,

* See Brugsch for translation of Smollett's letter; also Felsenstein.

shortness of breath, 'asthma', pains—all aggravated at times by 'a scorbutic affection'. Although he had retained his appetite, he had lost much weight. 'The nervous system is extremely irritable and subject to orgasms.' Bloodletting had only weakened him, while sea-bathing and the waters at Bath, had brought only temporary relief. Smollett's ideas about health and sickness were those of his time. The 'fibres' and 'vessels' of the human body were key elements. Physical activity benefitted them; contagion, climate and inactivity could have adverse effects. In his *Essay* he had stressed the importance of 'the preservation of their due tone and flexibility'.

Warm baths made 'rigid fibres more pliable and supple . . . enlarging the openings of the cuticular strainer' so that circulation and perspiration were improved. Unable to distinguish between symptoms, signs and states of disease, he could have had little idea of what, for example, would point to the tuberculous nature of a pulmonary complaint. Later, at Aix-en-Provence, he spoke of 'some kinds of pulmonary complaints such as tubercules, abscesses, or spitting of blood'. In his letter to Fizès, he attributed the relaxation of his own fibres to his sedentary mode of life; the closure of his pores had prevented the escape of humours.

The professor's eyes, he said, 'sparkled at sight of the fee'. Replying in French, which Smollett found 'extraordinary', his letter contained errors which suggested that he either could not understand Latin, or else that he had not read Smollett's letter carefully. Smollett was justifiably annoyed to be told that he had omitted his age, the duration of his illness, and had not said whether he suffered from cough, expectoration, loss of appetite, or whether his fever underwent exacerbations. 'In a word', said Fizès strangely, 'no detail has been entered into as to these matters'.

We can understand Smollett's disgust at all this, especially when he learned that the professor's diagnosis was pulmonary tuberculosis. He replied, in French, that he *had* provided the wanted information and that he could not be persuaded 'that there are any tubercules on my lung since I have never coughed pus'. The professor suggested that if his doubts persisted, he should come and see him, but he adhered to his diagnosis. Smollett refused this invitation and told Fizès that he now understood why he had enjoyed 'such a large share of reputation'. The treatment suggested—purging, broths, ass's milk, cough syrup (containing a dram of whalesperm)—and a diet which excluded meat, water-fowl, stews, salads, fruits and raw vegetables, we can safely assume would not have helped. Indeed, Smollett consoled himself a week later, *en route* to Nice, and took the advice of a village landlady, concerned about his health, who suggested plenty of *bouillon*, chicken, and white meat. She also told him to beware of Montpellier and its physicians.

THE ROAD TO NICE

Deciding to send on their baggage by sea to Villefranche, a coach and mules were hired, and the party left Montpellier on 13 November. It was cold and bright, the olives were as black as sloes, and the corn was already half a foot high. They crossed the Rhone on a bridge of boats at Buccaire, entering Provence, a pleasant, well cultivated countryside. The inns were not as good as those at Languedoc, but luckily did not possess those nasty conveniences on the top floor 'which an English traveller can very well dispense with'. At Nîmes, he recalled, a maid had told him that the French did not use the seat in 'the Temple of Cloacina', specially provided for the English, but 'left their offerings on the floor'.

At Brignolle he had a row with a landlady about the food she served up on fast day; and their coach broke an axle. They met the mistral, but were assured that it was usually short-lived and blew only a few times during the winter months. In the morning, nevertheless, the countryside was covered by a foot of snow, and the doctor thought he was back in the Scottish highlands.

At Muy, 'a wretched town', their coachmen would not proceed until the inn-keeper's account had been properly settled. Smollet disputed the cost, and went off searching for a magistrate. He brought one back to the inn—but had ultimately to pay up. 'I was obliged to travel in the night, in very severe weather, after all the fatigue and mortification I had undergone.'

Chastened by this experience perhaps, we find him, a few days later, sweetly advising travellers not to be mean with their money, for tipping made everything run smoother. 'Why', said he, in England, 'In one excursion of about two hundred miles my fellow traveller was in a passion . . . incessantly scolding either at landlords, landladies, waiters, hostlers, or postillions. We had bad horses, and bad chaises; set out from every stage with the curses of the people'—and managed to save little money. But Smollett himself, on his last journey from Bath to London, in heavy rain, began to tip handsomely 'out of pure compassion', thereby succeeding in obtaining 'elegant chaises with excellent horses' in which he sped along at great speed on wet roads.

At Fréjus, they caught a glimpse of the ruins of the Roman amphitheatre and aqueduct, and were 'treated with more politeness than we had met with in any other part of France'. Tipping?

At a post-house in the Esterel hills, in severe cold, the doctor had an unexpected and pleasurable surprise.

After dinner I chanced to look into another chamber that fronted the south, where the sun shone; and opening a window perceived, within a yard of my hand, a large tree loaded with oranges, many of which were ripe. You may judge what my astonishment was to find Winter in all his rigour reigning on one side of the house, and Summer in all her glory on the other.

Enchantment grew as they descended towards the sea.

This side of the hill is a natural plantation of the most agreable ever-greens, pines, firs, laurels, cypress, sweet myrtle, tamarisk, box and juniper, inters- persed with sweet marjoram, lavender, thyme, wild thyme, and sage.

They passed the night at Cannes, 'a little fishing town agreeably situated on the beach of the sea', journeying on next day, along the shore road, feeling 'as warm as it is in May in England', to Antibes. From there 'we had the first glimpse of Nice lying on the opposite side of the bay'.

NICE

Nice was to be their home for the next ten months; they spent the following winter in Italy, returning to Nice in the spring. They at first 'stewed a week in a paltry inn', then, while waiting for furniture in a house they rented, spent a short time in a house belonging to a helpful English consul. A suitable family apartment, Smollett discovered, could be obtained for an annual rent of about twenty pounds sterling. Their own lodgings comprised

a ground floor paved with brick, consisting of a kitchen, two large halls, a couple of good rooms with chimneys, three large closets that serve for bed-chambers and dressing rooms, a butler's room, and three apartments for servants, lumber or stores, to which we ascend by narrow stairs. I have likewise, two small gardens, well stocked with oranges, lemons, peaches, figs, grapes, corinths, sallad, and pot-herbs. It is supplied with a draw-well of good water, and there is another in the vestibule of the house, which is cool, large and magnificent.

They soon made friends and acquaintances among the English- speaking community and Smollett was interested to meet one consump- tive Englishman who had also consulted Professor Fizès at Montpellier. His prescription was identical with the one Smollett had received, but he was probably 'too far gone' to recover.

The rest and sunshine soon began to soothe Smollett's spirit, enough, at any rate, for him to mention that perhaps he had been too severe in his general comments about French people. He said that he felt no particular animosity towards them and that when he met a Frenchman worthy of his esteem, he had no difficulty in being cordial. He respected, also, the valour of military men; 'I have often heard it said that a French officer is generally an agreable companion when he is turned fifty'. Not that such benignity lasted long.

The town, which was not fortified, faced the sea, with a rampart and wall on its west side, and overhung on the east side by a rock on which stood the ruins of a castle. The countryside around resembled a garden, loaded with fruit and olive trees, and flowers of all kinds. He discovered that carnations were dispatched, 'one pressed upon another' in wooden boxes, to Turin, Paris, and sometimes even as far as London. The distant mountain peaks were white with snow. The country houses were white and square-shaped and there were some fine villas. Though enchanted with the rural scene, one thing he did miss; that was 'the song of a blackbird, thrush, linnet, goldfinch, or any other bird whatsoever'. It was the same throughout the south; 'scarce a sparrow, redbreast, tomtit, or wren can 'scape the guns and snares of those indefatigable fowlers'.

The population was about 12 000; the streets were narrow, the houses were built of stone, usually in three storeys, and had tiled roofs. The windows were usually filled with 'paper lozenges' but the bourgeois were beginning to have their houses 'sashed with glass'. Many had shutters, few had chimneys. A brazier of charcoal was sometimes used to heat a room. The fishermen hauled their boats up on the beach, but on the other side of the rock there was a small harbour, with a mole, and a garrison of soldiers. It was a free-port which attracted trade and contraband; it was usually full of small vessels from Sardinia, Spain, and Italy, loaded with salt, wine and other commodities. There was a lazarette, for quarantine purposes. Sardines and anchovies were salted, barreled, and exported widely. Tunny fishing was being developed; it was skilled and costly.

Wine and olive oil were in abundant supply. Grapes were pressed by naked feet in the vats, and when the juice was drawn off, squeezed again in a press. Fermentation was allowed to continue for up to twenty days and the wine was usually considered 'fit for drinking' in one month. Those who made their own wine chose grapes from different vineyards; peasant wine was often better than what could be purchased from a merchant. Mixed with water, Nice wine made an agreeable beverage; it was kept in casks, without corks, with a little oil at the top. It was not deemed worse for being left out of doors or for having been opened for a few days. In poor years there was a mischievous form of adulteration— the addition of 'the juice of pigeon's dung or quicklime, in order to give it a spirit which nature denied'.

Olives began to ripen and drop in November, but some remained on the trees until February and those were counted the most valuable. Before they began to fade and wrinkle they were ground with a mill-stone into a paste, which was subjected to a series of pressings. The oil was ladled into a vat half-filled with water; dirt fell to the bottom and the oil came to the top and was skimmed off. Some crude oil was extracted from the residue, and the dried pulp was used to burn as fuel.

The soil required careful watering and manuring. Cattle were few, dung from mules and asses was of little value; that from pigeons and man, was better. Smollett did not mention horses. 'Every peasant opens, at one corner of his wall, a public house of office for the reception of passengers; and in the town of Nice, every tenement is provided with one of these receptacles.' Peasants came collecting, with their asses and casks, before daylight. 'The jakes of a protestant family, who eat *gras* [meat] every day, bears a much higher price than the privy of a good catholic who lives *maigre* [fast-days or meat-less days] one half of the year. The vaults belonging to the convent of Minims [a monastic order] are not worth emptying.'

Olives, vines, fruit trees, and corn, crowded together on the stony terraces, looked stifled for want of room and air—such was the scarcity of land. But there were also pleasant adjacent meadows with excellent clover, wheat, rye and barley and oats—and splendid vegetables. In that winter there were potatoes, peas, asparagus, artichoke, cauliflower, beans, celery, endives, cabbage, radishes, turnips, carrots, sorrel, lettuce, onions, garlic, and shalot. There were mushrooms and truffles. In addition to the apples, pears, oranges and lemons, they enjoyed almonds, walnuts, chestnuts, filberts, medlars, and pomegranates. In the summer were strawberries, cherries, peaches, apricots and delicious water-melons. But the doctor found that at times, when he was hot and thirsty, there was really too much sweetness in these fruits and he did not care for the apples and pears. Most refreshing were the 'sorbettes'—iced froth made with the juices of oranges, apricots, or peaches'.

In the markets you could buy 'pretty good' beef, 'excellent pork and delicate lamb', but the mutton was indifferent. Chickens were scarce and pullets would not fatten, but the turkeys were good, and game such

as hare, partridge, quail, woodcock and snipe, was plentiful. Wild boar
had a delicious taste and the doctor thought it would make 'an excellent
barbecue'. There were few trout in the streams and the fish from the sea
were not as good as those from the ocean. Sole and flat-fish were few,
but there was ample mullet, dory, rock-fish, whiting, mackerel, and
excellent bass and '*moustel*'. Sword-fish was particularly esteemed, and
cuttle-fish stewed with onions was a popular dish. There were also the
tasty *écrivisse de mer* [cray-fish]. Bread, sardines, and anchovies were the
common staples of diet; 'nothing can be more delicious than fresh
anchovies fried in oil'.

Many things interested the sharp-eyed Smollett during his months in
Nice. He described the cultivation of the silkworm on mulberry leaves,
the Roman antiquities—the ruins of an amphitheatre, an underground
aqueduct, and vaults—and recorded some of the Latin inscriptions on
the remains. There were ten convents and three nunneries in the town,
so we hear his comments on the superstitions and ignorance of the local
faithful, and of the custom of seeking sanctuary in a church, and of feast
days and fast days. Among the ecclesiastics there, he heard of none who
had any learning. There was no intellectual life, no library, not even a
bookseller. He described the absurdities involved in the custom of
duelling, but noted that there was little crime. Drunkenness was
uncommon; one could walk out at night without fear. No one could wear
a dagger or carry a pistol; at night there was a curfew. Punishments were
severe—flagellation, service in a galley, the strappado, or hanging. In
strappado the condemned person was hauled up by the arms, which had
been tied behind his back, and dropped from a height, a few feet short of
the ground. This dislocated the shoulders; if repeated, the arms were
'rendered useless for life'.

In Villefranche he saw two Sardinian galleys with some two hundred
slaves aboard. He inspected one and was horrified at the filth and
wretched accommodation below decks. The prisoners were 'chained to
the banks on which they sit and row'. They only went to sea in the
summer; in harbour they were allowed to work, under guard. Barbary
corsairs terrorized the coastal towns and shipping, but Smollett thought
the galleys were useless. He was glad to hear that two English frigates
were on order.

Of the Nissards themselves, we are not surprised to hear that they had
their deficiencies. They spoke an uncouth patois, which was the 'ancient
Provencal, from which the Italian, Spanish, and French languages, have
been formed . . . the language that rose upon the ruins of the Latin
tongue' after the fall of the Roman Empire. The shopkeepers were

'generally poor, greedy and overreaching', the artisans were 'very lazy, very needy, very awkward, and void of all ingenuity'. Servants were 'slovenly, slothful, and unconscionable cheats'. Labourers were 'diminutive, meagre, withered, dirty and half-naked'. The poor peasants had no chance to improve themselves, oppressed, as they were, by mendicant friars and parish priests, as well as by their landlords.

The noblesse were as effete as those in Boulogne. 'Nice abounds in noblesse, marquisses, counts and barons. Of these, three or four families are really respectable.' The rest were sprung from the bourgeois; titles were purchased. There was one count whose father had sold macaroni in the street. They did not mix and Smollett never met them; the local English consul had lived in the country for thirty-four years 'without having once eat or drank in any of their houses'. Most of the females were 'pot-bellied' which he attributed to the large amounts of 'vegetable trash' which they consumed. They strolled around together, with their mistresses and gigolos. 'The husband and the *cicisbeo* [gigolo] live together as sworn brothers; and the wife and the mistress embrace each other with marks of the warmest affection.' But he discovered that this Italian fashion was common among all ranks of people in Nice. 'There is not such a passion as jealousy known.'

But it was in search of health that Smollett came to Nice and he left an account of its climate, based on his carefully kept 'register of the weather'. In due course it served to bring about the introduction of the English to the French Riviera, promoting Nice as a resort. A hundred years later, despite his remarks about the French, we find his name, albeit spelled incorrectly as 'Smolet', on a street sign in the town.

He explained that the town was screened from the north by the maritime alps and that there was less wind and rain there 'than in any other part of the world that I know'. The air was serene; for months on end there was nothing above you but a blue sky. In December and January, it was true, there were winds and rain; in the spring there were showers, and in the summer, the occasional storm. But in general, the dry heat and the light breezes were all that could be desired. He found that he could breathe more freely, he had fewer colds and his spirits were more alert. He began to bathe in the sea in May, being carried there in a sedan-chair. Some Swiss soldiers tried it, then a few Nissards. He thought some tents on the beach could be erected.

But he was not well. He continued to lose weight and he thought he had scurvy. There was a recurring rash on the back of one hand, swelling of his gums, and pains in his joints, but it is difficult to understand why he should become scorbutic on a diet which contained so much fresh fruit and vegetables. Yet his years in the navy had made the disease familiar, although he thought it was climatic in origin. He was seemingly unaware of what his fellow Scot, James Lind, had written about it in 1753, after his own years as a naval surgeon. But, then, the admiralty order enjoining the use of lemon juice was not made until 1795.

There were drawbacks in Nice, he wished the English to know about. In the summer you could only escape from the swarms of flies and midges by getting under your mosquito net; there were also fleas and bugs. Other deficiencies were the lack of shaded walks, and carriages. He actually advised valetudinarians to winter in Nice and go up into the hills for the summer. He himself contemplated going up to a little town called Rocabiliare, twenty-five miles inland, where he understood the waters were 'attenuating and deobstruent, consequently of service in disorders arising from a languid circulation, a viscidity of the juices, a lax fibre and obstructed viscera'. But, poor man, he decided on a sea voyage to Italy, and in any case, he had 'a most eager curiosity to see the antiquities of Florence and Rome', adding that 'a sea voyage has been found of wonderful efficacy in consumptive cases'. Was he accepting Fizès diagnosis?

BY SEA TO LERICI

To journey to Italy over the mountains would have been far too strenuous and the road along the coast was fit only for mules and foot passengers. 'What a pity it is, he said, 'that they cannot restore the celebrated *Via Aurelia* . . . which extended from Rome by way of Genoa, and through this country as far as Arles'. So 'a gondola' was hired, rowed by four men and steered by the owner, and he set off at the beginning of September with his wife, Miss C——, Mr R—— a native of Nice, and one servant. They went on board at ten in the morning, putting into Monaco about noon, where a toll had to be paid. The small town stood upon a rock and had a romantic appearance; the palace was elegant and the fortifications in good repair. The Prince was a Frenchman who had married the heiress of Monaco, whose name was Grimaldi.

They passed Menton and Ventimiglia in the afternoon and spent the night at an inn at St. Remo where they 'fared villainously'. They had to remain there the next day as a high wind had sprung up, but they enjoyed the company of a jolly Franciscan monk and a maestro of the spinet. The women of St. Remo were handsome, with good eyes and 'open ingenuous countenances'. On the following day they got as far as the town of Moli, where the inn was even worse than that at St. Remo; bugs drove the doctor from his bed and he slept on a chest, wrapped in a greatcoat. They could get no milk there, although there were plenty of goats about; he wondered why goat's milk was not used for children. They arrived at Genoa about five in the afternoon of the fourth day, passing the famous lighthouse, and entering the harbour between two long moles, mounted with brass cannon. So well were they entertained at their inn, that they decided to spend a few days there.

It was not without reason that Genoa was called 'La Superba'. It was a stately city which had the 'face of business'. The streets were busy, the shops and markets were well-stocked and the bread was the best and whitest he had ever tasted. There were two streets which were lined on each side with 'palaces adorned with gardens and fountains'.* They visited some palaces and churches, but there was more magnificence than taste in some of the latter. The cathedral was gothic and gloomy and he was unimpressed by the Ponte Carignano, but from a nearby church they had a fine view of the city, the sea, and the surrounding countryside, which looked like 'a continent of groves and villas'.

Through the kindness of a Genoese lady, who was 'one of the most intelligent and best-bred persons' he had known in any country, they met people of education and culture. One of them 'knew me by reputation'. Smollett was concerned about the state of the Genoese Republic, and he commented on its trade, security and prospects. They were then under the protection of the French, but with English supremacy in the Mediterranean, it would be wise if they sought our assistance.

A few days later they went off in the same boat, passing by several pretty towns and villages, Portofino and Lavagno, to reach Sestri Levante, where they spent a night of discomfort in an inn owned by a butcher. He had 'the looks of an assassin' and a wife who was 'a great masculine virago, who had all the air of having frequented the slaughterhouse'. He was glad to escape with his 'throat uncut'. The coastline was barren next day until they rounded Portovenere and entered the bay of Spezia, where plantations of olives and oranges delightfully surrounded them. The former naval surgeon observed that it would make 'an admirable station for a British squadron'. That night, in the post-house at Lerici, he slept on four chairs, with a portmanteau

* 'When shall I forget the Streets of Palaces; the Strada Nuova and the Strada Balbi!', exclaimed Charles Dickens in Genoa in 1844 (*Pictures from Italy*). Strada Nuova became Via Garibaldi in 1882.

for a pillow, as the place assigned him was too close and confined. They went on by road to Pisa the next day, arriving about eight in the evening, and finding 'a very good inn'.

PISA

Here was a fine old city, quiet, dignified, with open well-paved streets (some alas with grass agrowing), churches of taste, and with people who were reputedly sociable and polite. On each side of the river Arno, as it ran through the city, there was 'a beautiful wharf of freestone'. But the city itself was rather desolate, the university was 'much decayed' and there were only 'a few men of taste and learning'. The population was only 16 000, whereas when it was the capital of a flourishing and powerful republic, it was a 'noble' city of some 150 000. Nevertheless, he preferred it to the tumult of a populous commercial city.

The Campanile, or 'hanging tower', was 'a beautiful cylinder of eight stories, each adorned with a round of columns, rising one above another'. A plummet dropped from the top, 188 feet high, would fall sixteen feet outside its base. The inclination was clearly not planned, as some had claimed, as one could see how the pillars on one side had sunk into the ground. The same subsidence explained the leaning towers to be seen in Bologna, Venice, and Ravenna.

At the cathedral, with its 'great number of massy pillars of porphyry, granite, jasper, giullo and verde antico' (antique yellow and green marble), what caught his eye were the bronze doors ('brass gates'), embossed with panels illustrating scenes from the old and new testaments. He said, 'I was so charmed with this work, that I could have stood a whole day to examine and admire it'. The path by the frescoes in the cemetery of Campo Santo was 'a noble walk for a contemplative philosopher'. The adjacent hospital was large and elegant.

FLORENCE

The road to Florence, along the banks of the muddy Arno, took them through hills and vales, woods, and waters which reminded him of Middlesex and Hampshire—but for the vines about the trees. In Italy they did not prop their vines on sticks in rows, but twined them round the hedgerow trees, which they covered with their fruit and leaves. More space was thus left in which to grow grass and corn.

Florence still retained the marks of a majestic capital, with its piazzas and palaces, statues and fountains, and its arcades and bridges. The

Smolletts lodged with an English lady, near the river. There were many English residents and visitors, as it was considered 'a must' on the Grand Tour. Horace Walpole had spent a year there. Edward Gibbon was there that very summer, going on to Rome in the autumn, where on 15 October, he described, twenty-five years later, he was inspired to write his book, 'while musing amidst the ruins of the Capitol'. An Englishman called Acton, a former sea captain, was an 'admiral' in the Tuscan Navy, and Smollett observed that the tomb of an English soldier from Essex, who had served in the Florentine Army, could be seen in the cathedral.

The Florentine noblesse were not inclined to receive foreign visitors without titles, so he found it strange that they were not above selling their figs and wine from their houses. Outside each was a knocker and a flask to signify their intention. A titled family would not permit a daughter to marry into an untitled one—not even if it was a distinguished professional family. Tuscan speech was disagreeably guttural and when the doctor first heard it he thought the person had lost his palate, through some 'misfortune in the course of his amours'. Opera and poetry were popular, but what Florentines really enjoyed was church pageantry. In a procession he saw, there were the noblesse, girls from an institution wearing violet gowns and white veils, and penitents in sackcloth, and monks 'bawling and bellowing the litanies'. Many of the so-called penitents were hired for the occasion and took care to protect themselves from the scourging by wearing 'secret armour, either women's bodice, or quilted jackets'.

Smollett said he did not wish to burden his readers with accounts of everything they could see in Florence. One German writer had been 'so laboriously circumstantial in his descriptions, that I could never peruse them without suffering the headache, and recollecting the old observation, that the German genius lies more in the back than in the brain'. He came to be criticized for the way in which he disparaged so much classical art, but in Florence he did admit that he was not setting himself up as a judge in such matters. 'I am used to speak my own mind freely on all subjects that fall under the cognizance of the senses; though I must freely own, there is something more than common sense required to discover and distinguish the more delicate beauties of painting'.

Across 'the covered bridge' from the Pitti Palace there was that 'famous gallery' (the Uffizi) through which, he said, he would walk each day if he were resident in the city. It was finer than 'the Lycaeum, the groves of Academus, or any porch or philosophical alley in Athens or Rome'. The profusion of display in this celebrated museum bewildered the imagination—statues, busts, pictures, medals, marquetry, cabinets, jewels, and ancient arms and military machines. Of the marble statues, he admired Leda with the Swan (Tintoretto's painting is also there), Aesculapius, the head of Alexander the Great, the kneeling Narcissus, and the two Bacchi. He did not enjoy looking at the statue of the hermaphrodite, 'no other than a monster in nature', and although he admired the limbs and proportions of the Venus Pontia, 'commonly called de Medicis', he thought her features were not beautiful, and her attitude awkward. What he most appreciated was the statue of a slave, 'called the Whetter'. The slave was kneeling, whetting a knife, and was supposed to have just heard talk of a conspiracy; 'I never saw such an expression of anxious attention, as appears on his countenance'.

Among the paintings at the Uffizi, he was most charmed with the Venus by Titian (Venus of Urbino) with 'its sweetness of expression and tenderness of colouring'. At the Pitti, surprisingly, the best-loved of Raphael's madonnas—the Madonna of the Chair—did not wholly satisfy him. Although it was 'gay, agreable, and very expressive of maternal tenderness', he thought it was 'defective in dignity and sentiment'. The madonna had 'the expression of a peasant', an observation which the present writer at first dismissed, but which still puzzles him.

The famous bronze doors ('brass gates') of the Baptistery—'the Gates of Paradise' (said Michelangelo)—were viewed with pleasure, but he still preferred those at Pisa. The cathedral was 'remarkable for nothing but its cupola', and the chapel of St. Lorenzo, 'a monument of ill taste and extravagance'.

AND SO TO ROME

On the road to Rome, by way of Siena, Montefiascone, and Viterbo, in a coach hired for seven weeks, they experienced two mishaps. At one point a wheel came off, and at another, two of their horses fell, and almost strangled themselves as they lay struggling in the harness. Smollett, furious with the hostler who had, he said, provided two, young unbroken horses because he had not been tipped, rounded up a local magistrate, made the customary accusations and vowed to report the incident to the British minister in Florence. 'Of all the people I have ever seen, the hostlers, postillions, and other fellows hanging about the posthouses in Italy, are the most greedy, impertinent, and provoking.'

When they reached the Roman Campagna he was filled with 'pity and indignation' that such an ancient stretch of cultivated land should have been allowed to wither and decay. He could not understand why the marshes were not drained for they polluted the summer air with their 'putrid exhalations'. The castle of St. Angelo was one of the first objects to catch the eye of the visitor, and 'however ridiculous as a fortress' it was nevertheless 'respectable as a noble monument of antiquity'.

They entered the city by the Porta del Populo—'an august entrance'—with its noble piazza, obelisk, fountain, and churches. They secured comfortable lodgings in the Piazza d'Espagna, where the English liked to reside, and furnishing themselves with books and maps, they procured a guide and hired a town-coach. The English there were already accustomed to leaving visiting cards with new arrivals from home; 'they expected to have the visit returned the next day, when they give orders not to be at home'. This particular refinement was one 'which the English have invented by the strength of their own genius, without any assistance from France, Italy or Lapland'.

Nothing was more agreeable to the eyes of a stranger, he wrote, than the many ornamented fountains in the city, with their 'prodigious quantities of cool, delicious water' brought in by the aqueducts of the ancient Romans, and so wisely restored by beneficent popes. There were said to have been fourteen, some bringing water from a distance of forty miles, and wide enough to admit an armed horseman. They were fortified and blocked up when besieging Goths cut off the water, and subsequently fell into ruin. In the architecture of modern Rome he looked in vain for 'that simplicity of grandeur, those large masses of light and shadow' which so characterized the buildings of classical antiquity. Now, there was crowding inside and outside the churches and palaces, so that the design was effectively destroyed by the assemblage of 'pretty ornaments which distract the eye' and fill up the interior, while outside, proportions were concealed and outlines hidden.

The gardens of the Pincio and the Villa Borghese, with their fine views and long avenues among the pines, shrubs and flowers, so favoured by the people of Rome, he found disappointing. In such a fine, landscaped park an Englishman expected things to be 'inter-mixed with an agreeable negligence . . . and rural simplicity'. Fountains might be sculpturally elegant but the water they spouted could be more naturally conveyed in 'little rivulets and streams to refresh the thirsty soil' or managed in cascades. Here was a garden that did not compare with that in Stowe in Buckinghamshire. The Italians understood art but not the beauties of nature.

Following a conversation with an Italian expatiating upon the greatness and wealth of modern Rome, Smollett thought that the popes would do well 'to avoid misunderstandings with the maritime protestant states, especially the English', as Rome's defences were poor and the city could be taken without difficulty by landing an army a dozen miles away.

But it was Ancient Rome that he had come to see and he went down to the Forum and began to recall lines from Horace and Livy, Virgil and Ovid, Tacitus, and Juvenal. He walked down the Capitoline hill, past pillars and pedestals and 'shafts stuck in rubbish', through the triumphal arch of Septimius Severus, past the Emperor Vespasian's temple, to the Arch of Constantine and on to the Colosseum. 'I suppose', he mused, 'there is more concealed below ground than appears above'. The stones of the Colosseum had been used by popes and princes to build and adorn their 'paltry palaces' and even the miserable peasants' houses had walls and gardens full of 'shafts and capitals of marble columns, heads, arms, legs, mutilated trunks of statues'. Enough of the Colosseum remained, however, 'to convey a very sublime idea of ancient magnificence'. Thoughts of the bloody scenes which had been enacted there prompted him to comment on the difference between bravery and savagery; 'Some of this sanguinary spirit is inherited by the inhabitants of a certain island that shall be nameless—but, mum for that'.

The Pantheon was 'no more that a plain unpierced cylinder, or circular wall, with two fillets and a cornice, having a vaulted roof or cupola, open in the centre'—reminding him, to the disgust of Sterne, of 'a huge cockpit'. Although he admired the construction of the ancient circuses and arenas, some of which could be flooded, he thought that Roman horsemanship and oarsmanship could have been nothing to boast about. The Circus Maximus was not as long as the Mall; St. James's Park was a better place to race, and if a Roman had seen the track at Newmarket his eyes would have been opened. The Caracalla circus 'scarce affords breathing room for an English hunter'. And as for the mock naval battles—the Naumachia—'How would a British sailor relish an advertisement that a mock engagement between two squadrens of men-of-war would be exhibited on such a day in the serpentine at Hyde Park?'. Why flood artificial basins with fresh water when there was the Tiber, and a few miles away, the sea. Their galleys were probably no bigger than some fishing-smacks. 'I do believe in my conscience that half a dozen English frigates would have been able to defeat both the contending fleets at the famous battle of Actium . . . an event that decided the fate of an empire.'

Doctor Smollett recalled that bathing had become so habitual for Romans, that Galen had mentioned a philosopher who immediately

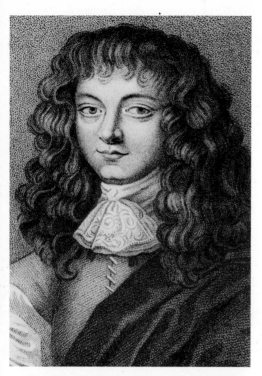

1. Edward Browne.

2. On the Danube below Passau (from Browne).

3. St. Stephen's Cathedral, Vienna. The Turkish star and crescent above the Christian Cross on the steeple (from Browne).

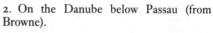

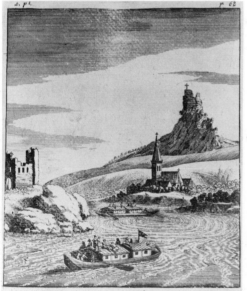

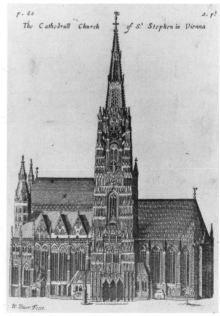

2.

3.

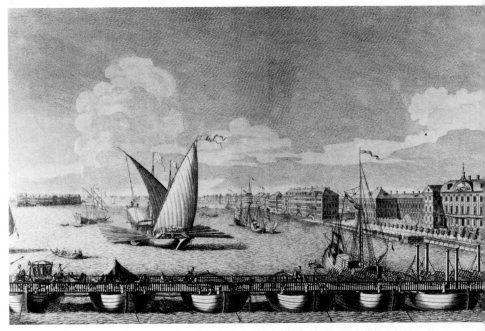

4. Leningrad, a view after Makhayev, 1753. The river Neva and the bridge of boats.

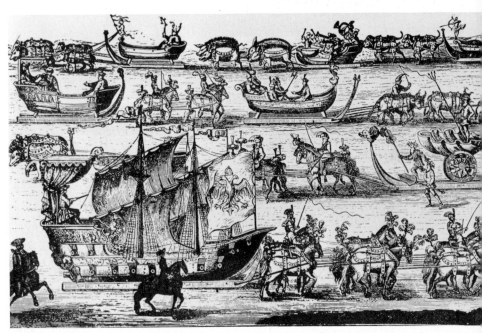

5. *Moscow, 1722: the Royal procession.* This gargantuan masquerade was witnessed by Bell. It was held to celebrate victory over the Swedes and to demonstrate the success of the new Russian fleet of Peter the Great. For days on end, animals of all kinds drew vessels through the streets.

6. Alexander Hamilton of the 'Ancient & Honourable Tuesday Club', a self-caricature.

7. The first page of Hamilton's original manuscript.

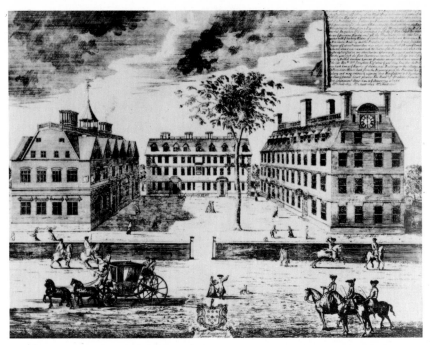

8. Harvard College, Cambridge, Mass., Wm. Burgis 1725–26. It had 'a handsome clock, a good bell, a large courtyard, and a library of 3 or 4 thousand volumes'. The clock is still there, on Massachusetts Hall.

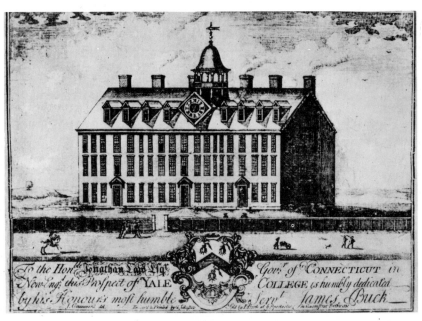

To the Hon.ble Jonathan Law Esq.r Gov.r of Connecticut in New Eng.d this Prospect of Yale College is humbly dedicated by his Honour's most humble serv.t James Buch

9. Yale College, New Haven, Conn., the earliest known view, J. Greenwood, 1749. 'A wooden building 200 foot long and three stories high, in the middle of which is a little cupola with a clock upon it.'

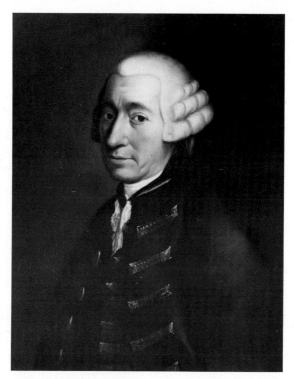

10. Tobias Smollett, by an unknown artist, *c.* 1770.

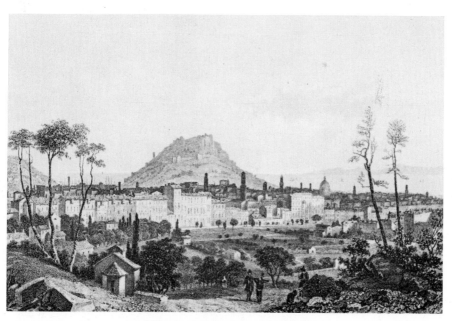

11. Nice, from a contemporary engraving.

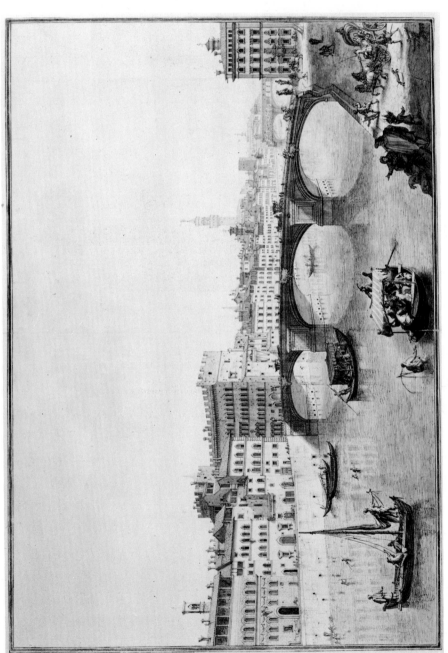

12. Florence. The river Arno and the Ponte Santa Trinita, by G. Zocchi.

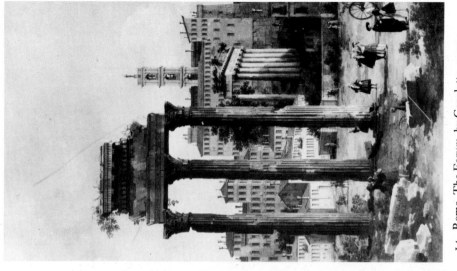

14. Rome. The Forum, by Canaletto, 1742.
'I suppose there is more concealed below ground than appears above.'

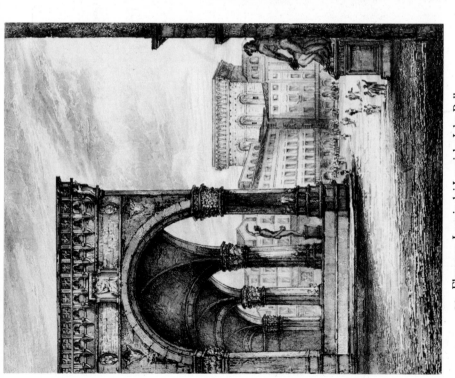

13. Florence. Loggia dei Lanzi, by John Bell.

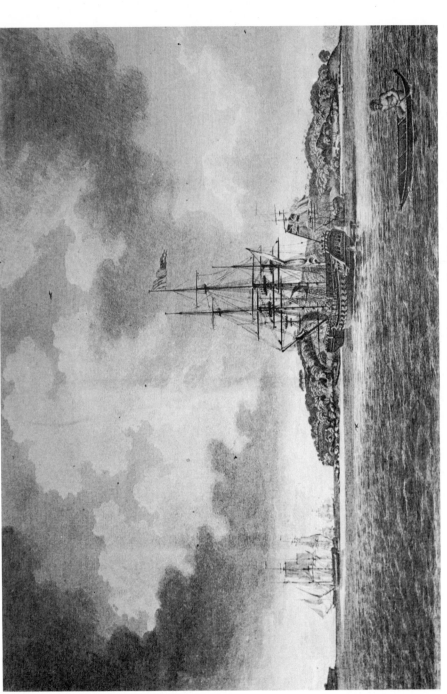

15. The frigate HMS *Sirius* and the sloop HMS *Supply* in Botany Bay. (From Phillip's *Voyage*, 1789.)

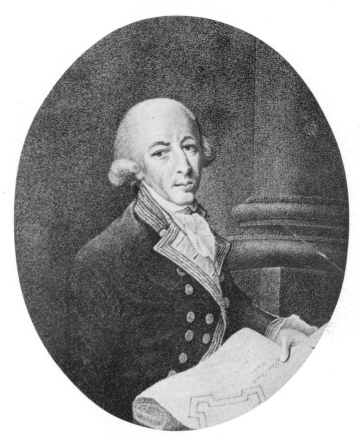

16. Captain Arthur Phillip, commander of the
First Fleet and first Governor of New South
Wales. (From Phillip's *Voyage*, 1789.)

DORSET
ANY PERSON WILFULLY INJURING
ANY PART OF THIS COUNTY BRIDGE
• WILL BE GUILTY OF FELONY AND •
UPON CONVICTION LIABLE TO BE
TRANSPORTED FOR LIFE
BY THE COURT
7 & 8 GEO 4 C 30 S 13 ❀ T FOOKS

17. A plaque which may be seen in the Dorset County Museum,
Dorchester. (Photograph by the author.)

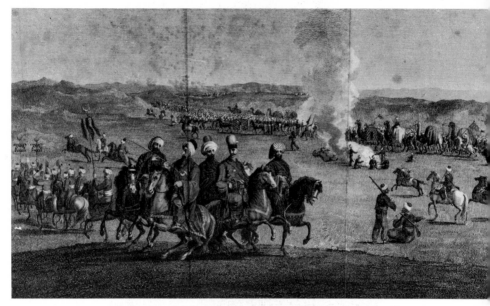

18. The Grand Vizier's army *en route* from Jaffa to Cairo (from Wittman).

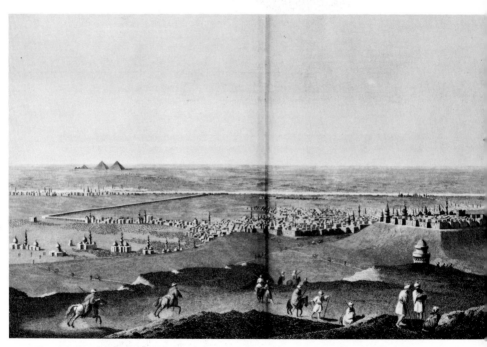

19. Cairo, as depicted by D. V. Denon, one of Bonaparte's artists in Egypt. (From *Voyage dans la Bas. Haute Egypte pendant les campagnes de Bonaparte en 1798 et 1799*, 2 vols, London (1807).)

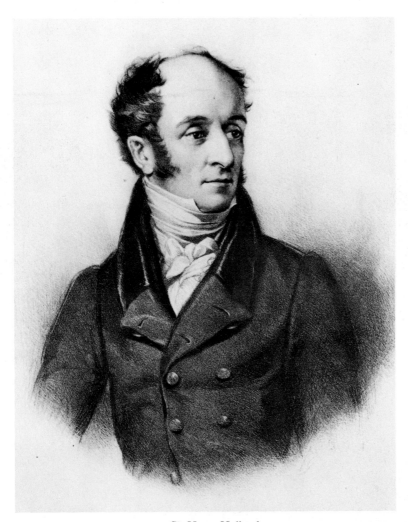

20. Sir Henry Holland.

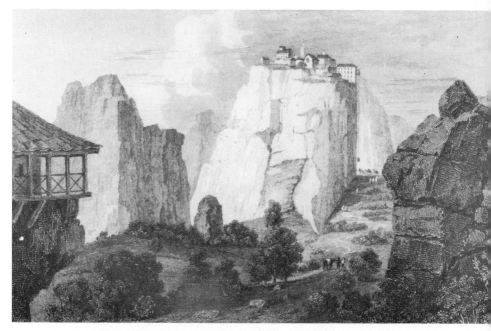

21. Meteora (from Holland).

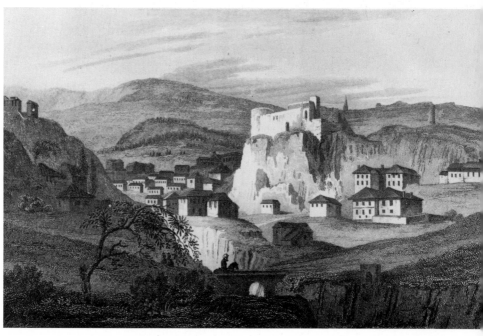

22. The castle at Gjinokaster, fifteen miles south of Tepelene (from Holland).

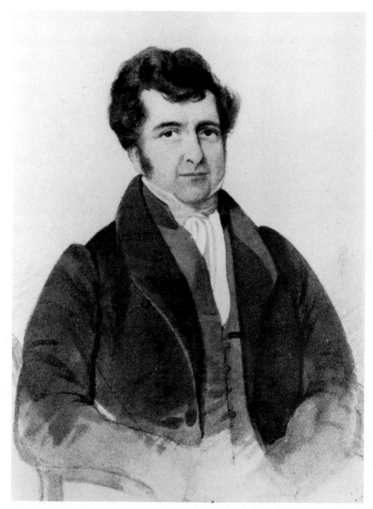

23. Richard Bright.

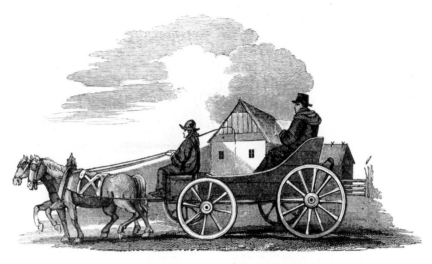

24. Hungarian post-travelling (from Bright).

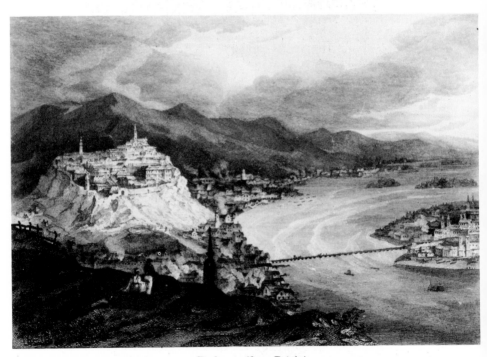

25. Budapest (from Bright).

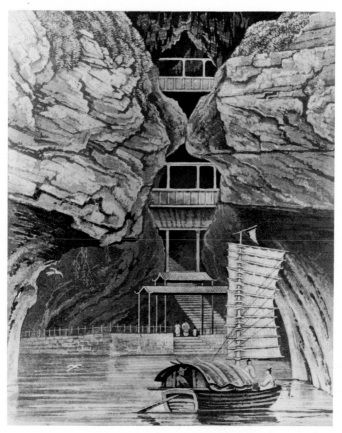

26. A Chinese riverside temple (from Abel).

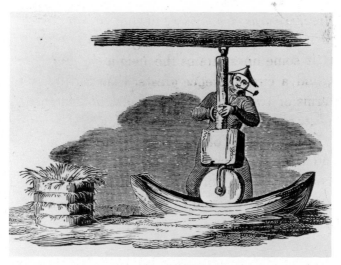

27. Machine for extracting oil. Seeds are ground in an iron-lined, canoe-shaped tree trunk, by a weighted wheel suspended from a beam. Man moves wheel to and fro (from Abel).

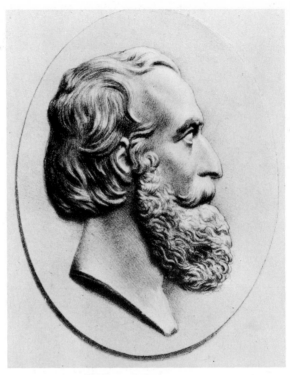

28. Thomas Hodgkin from the frontispiece of his book,
1866.

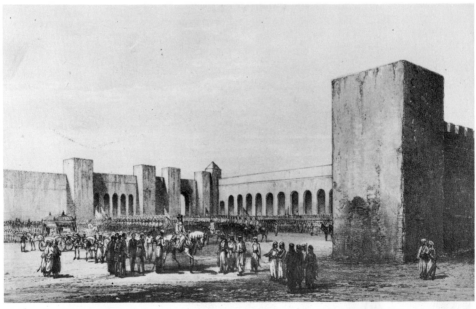

29. The Sultan of Morocco, on his white horse, in Marrakesh. Sir Moses Montefiore reads his
address, while others (including a bearded gentleman who is probably Hodgkin) stand behind him,
on the left.

went down with fever if he omitted his daily visit to the baths. The time for bathing was from noon till evening; there were separate places for the sexes but no distinction was made between patrician and plebeian. Some were free, in others you paid. The baths of Caracalla could accommodate 2300 at one time and were 'adorned with all the charms of painting, architecture and sculpture . . . the pipes conveying the water were of silver'. They did use cool water in summer but otherwise prefered it milk-warm and perfumed; scented ointments were used in the vapour-baths. But this luxuriation must have 'tended to debilitate the fibres already too much relaxed by the heat of the climate'. A plunge into the Tiber would have been more beneficial. Within the *thermae* various places were assigned for different activities; the *basilicae*, where bathers assembled; the *nationates*, for swimming; the *portici*, for walking and conversation; the *atria*, or courts; the *ephibia*, for exercise; the *frigidaria*, where there were cooling draughts of air; the *gymnasia*, where poets, orators, and philosophers recited their works; and all around were groves and walks and stone seats. The whole controlled by rules and under the supervision of a censor. You feel that Dr Smollett would have been at home there.

Despite all this, the doctor concluded that the city must have been a crowded and dirty place, with the Tiber 'the general receptacle of the *cloaca maxima* and all the filth of Rome'. One year, the collected cobwebs alone weighed ten thousand pounds! The Romans had some strange domestic habits. One was 'the delicate custom of taking vomits at each other's houses, when they were invited to dinner'. Another was the abominable practice of swaddling infants, which he saw depicted in a statue, and had first seen in a foundling hospital in Paris. It resulted in obstruction of the circulation, compression of the limbs and brain and was no doubt responsible for the bandy legs, small bodies, and large hydrocephalic heads which were so common in the south of France and in Italy. All nonsense of course.

Assuring his readers that he had not seen one half of all the art treasures of Rome, he avowed that he had described nothing that he had not seen. He did not profess to have 'the nice discernment and delicate sensibility of the true connoisseur' but had tried to give his personal impression of some of the most celebrated pieces'.

There was the bronze ('Corinthian brass') equestrian statue of Marcus Aurelius in the Capitoline piazza which greatly pleased him; the splendid elegance and accurate anatomy of the Dying Gladiator (Dying Gaul) where 'you may count all the spines of the vertebrae' and admire the course of the muscles (including the 'longissimi dorsi') and the softness of the flesh; the group known as The Farnese Bull, mentioned by Pliny, depicted 'such spirit, ferocity and indignant resistance' as he had never previously seen on canvas or in stone, as Pliny had thought, but it surpassed his expectation. The piazza of St. Peter's was 'altogether sublime' but the church itself would have been a masterpiece, 'entire and perfect' if it stood alone, detached from the irregular mass of Vatican buildings in its rear.

If he had been the owner of Raphael's Transfiguration he would have cut it in two parts 'as the three figures in the air attract the eyes so strongly, that little or no attention is paid to those below in the mountain'. He was struck by 'the expression of dignity on the face of Christ . . . and by the suprising lightness of the figure, that hovers like a beautiful exhalation in the air'. He did not mention the 'epileptic' child in the foreground. A Titian virgin, and The Judgement of Paris he admired. But Michelangelo, 'with all his skill in anatomy, his correctness of design, his grand composition, his fire and force of expression, seems to have very little idea of grace'. In The Pietà, the emaciation of the figure of Christ made it look as if 'he had died of consumption'. It was a disease never far from his mind. But who could agree with him that there was 'something indelicate, not to say indecent', in the picture of 'a man's body, stark naked, lying upon the knees of a woman'. His mind could take the strangest turns. He watched some mosaic artists at work, admired their ingenuity, and learned that the number of the drawers in which they kept their colours, went up to seventeen thousand.

'The implements of popish superstition' he found most disagreeable. 'What a pity it is', he said, 'that the labours of painting should have been so much employed on the shocking subjects of martyrology'. There were numberless pictures of flagellation, decapitation and crucifixion, not to mention Stephen battered with stones, Sebastian stuck full of arrows, Laurence frying upon the coals, and Bartholomew flayed alive. All an encouragement to 'a spirit of religious fanaticism'. We feel he was genuinely nauseated.

When speaking of the appreciation of art in general, he said that English people, 'the moment they set foot in Italy, they are seized with the ambition of becoming connoisseurs'. Dealers in antiques were there to snare them with 'trash'. The inexperienced could easily be 'bubbled by a knavish antiquarian'. He thought that ancient Romans had possessed taste enough to admire the arts of Greece, but had not themselves produced any celebrated painter or sculptor. 'Like the English of this day, they made a figure in poetry, history, and ethics; but the excellence of painting, sculpture, architecture, and music, they never could attain.' One wonders what he would think today.

One curious point may be mentioned. He said that the population of ancient Rome was about 'seven millions' (it was not more than two). He also said, when writing of English travellers, that he had seen 'a boy of seventy-two, now actually travelling through Italy, for improvement, under the auspices of another boy of twenty-two'. (I have seen this quoted in references to oldsters, not youngsters, foot-loose in Italy.) Are we dealing with misprints? It is possible that in both instances he had written the numeral '2' and it was misread as '7' so that we read of 7 million instead of 2, and 72 instead of 22.

RETURN TO NICE

Our tetchy xenophobic doctor, anxious to see the cascade at Terni, decided to return to Florence through the hills of Umbria, by way of Narni, Spoleto, and Perugia. He was assured that the route was shorter, easier and safer, and that it was served by 'exceeding good auberges'. But knowing our traveller by now, we are not surprised to learn that it was in all respects, very much otherwise. It was, or at any rate reads, like a week of torment. The way lay over 'steep mountains', by 'precipices', through rain and mud along narrow stony roads, and—'as for the public houses, they are in all respects the most execrable that I ever entered'. Landlords, coachmen, and hostlers were rascals; 'I repeat it again; of all the people I ever knew, the Italians are the most villainously rapacious'.

There was some enjoyment. The cascade at Termi was 'an object of tremendous sublimity'; there were some pleasant green valleys, the beautiful Lake Trasimene, and views of small towns and villages perched on the summits of hills, the most striking of which was Assisi.

But even at Termi one had to stand on 'the brink of a precipice' and the view was too oblique. There were numerous delays; a wheel was lost—an iron on the coach gave way—horses were not available—and on mountain roads they had to get out and walk. On one hill the horses were so exhausted that their carriage started to roll backwards 'to the very edge of a precipice'. They were only saved from being 'dashed to pieces' when a passer-by thrust a stone under a wheel. At the inn in Foligno, Smollett was choosing a bedroom and found one was locked. He was told that 'a filthy beast' had just died there and it had not yet been made ready. He enquired about the nature of 'the beast', and the Landlord informed him that it was 'an English heretic'. The doctor must have been tired that evening, as he says nothing of any fracas, consoling himself the following day when he learned that he had been mistaken for a German catholic. At another inn they had to cook their own supper, and ran the risk of being devoured by rats. After one bad night he was seized with 'a dangerous fit of hooping-cough, which terrified my wife, alarmed my company, and brought the whole community into the house'.

On the seventh evening, as they neared Florence, they experienced their severest trial. Rejecting the advice of their coachman, 'an impertinent rascal' who claimed that the road was broken up by two days of rain, and also of the 'ruffian' of a keeper of the last inn which they had inspected and found unfit, Smollett and his wife decided to push on to the ferry across the Arno a few miles below Florence. Miss C—— and Mr ——, their companions from Nice, rested at the inn. The ferry boat could not accommodate their coach so they had to tramp the three miles to the city, guided by a man carrying their boxes.

The night was dark and wet; the road slippery and dirty; not a soul was seen, nor a sound was heard; all was silent, dreary and horrible. I laid my account with a violent fit of illness from the cold I should infallibly catch, if I escaped assassination, the fears of which were the more troublesome as I had no weapon to defend our lives. While I laboured under the weight of my greatcoat which made the streams of sweat flow down my face and shoulders, I was plunging in the mud, up to the mid-leg at every step; and obliged at the same time to support my wife, who wept in silence, half dead with terror and fatigue. To crown our vexation, our conductor walked so fast that he was often out of sight, and I imagined he had run away with the boxes. All I could do, on these occasions, was to hollow as loud as I could, and swear horribly that I would blow his brains out. I did not know but that these oaths and menaces might keep other rogues in awe. In this manner did we travel three long miles, making an almost intire circuit of the city wall, without seeing the face of a human creature, and at length reached the gate, where we were examined by the guard, and allowed to pass, after they told us it was a long mile from thence to the house of Vanini, where we proposed to lodge . . . It was nearly ten at night, when we entered the auberge in such a draggled and miserable condition, that Mrs Vanini almost fainted at sight of us, on the supposition that we had met with some terrible disaster, and that the rest of the company were killed.

But at midnight their companions arrived safely, and in the morning, their coach and baggage; 'when all of us found ourselves well refreshed, and in good spirits'.

After a short stay in Florence they journeyed back through Pisa to Lerici, but were delayed there a couple of nights by the weather, before sailing to Genoa. On the beach at Lerici there was a solitary Englishman who took some care to avoid them, although he knew they were English. His valet informed Smollett's servant that 'in coming through France, his master had travelled three days in company with two other English gentlemen, whom he met upon the road, and in all that time he never spoke a word to either'. This, said Smollett, was 'a character truly British'.*

At Sestri Levante, their butcher-landlord had his house in better order and was much more obliging, which favourable change the Dr attributed to a certain 'humility and submission' induced by the havoc wrought in his olive grove by a recent storm. They were in Genoa the next day, and after a night at Finale, where the inn-keeper was another 'assassin', they sailed on, but were driven by high winds to take shelter in Porto Maurizio. In its post-house was a girl with 'the confluent smallpox', in a room through which they had to pass; the smell was so strong that it perfumed the whole house.

Taking to mules at this place, they set off on the fifteen mile journey to St. Remo—'and a very ridiculous cavalcade we formed' with the ladies having to sit astride. It took them seven hours, on a narrow road 'along one continued precipice'. At St. Remo their old lodgings were 'whitewashed and in great order'. The boat came round from Porto Maurizio on the next morning and carried them on to Nice by 'about four in the afternoon'.

He felt that his two months in Italy, despite the hardships endured, 'the continued agitation', and 'the violent fits of passion' he had suffered, had done him no harm. In fact, he felt braced up and stronger, attributing this to the beneficial effects of exceptional physical exertion. During the months of November and December, he felt in 'good health and spirits' and was able to stand for two hours in a cold gallery of Nice Cathedral where he went to hear high mass on Christmas Eve—out of 'curiosity', of course.

NICE: THE SECOND WINTER

He now felt able to comment in a general way about the climate in Nice. It was exceptionally wet that winter, raining on fifty-six days during the four months from November to March. If he came again he would spend the summer months in Grasse, among the hills of Provence, and famed for its perfumes. But the contrast between the English and French agricultural scene impressed him forcibly. He recalled the

* In Kinglake's *Eothen*, again it was the servants who induced the two shy Englishmen to halt their camels, turn back, and exchange a few words in the middle of the Sinai desert.

richness of the former, with its solid farmhouses, fine herds and rich crops, and the tall, stout peasants. In France the fields were unfenced, cattle and horses were few, the farmhouses mean and the peasants undernourished; 'I cannot help thinking they groan under oppression'. There was 'a violent fermentation of different principles' astir; 'a spirit of freedom takes the ascendant'. The king should undertake major reforms—in taxation, rural economy, and in controlling the extravagances which were to be seen everywhere. 'A French general in the field is always attended by thirty or forty cooks; and thinks it is incumbent upon him, for the glory of France, to give a hundred dishes every day at his table.' In one military headquarters at Nice, 'there were fifty scullions constantly employed in the great square in plucking poultry'. If nothing was done to improve matters 'the influence of the commons will insensibly encroach upon the pretensions of the crown'.

In February he went with his servant, over the mountains, by mule, to Turin, a distance of some ninety miles. *En route*, they joined up with a Nice acquaintance, a Marquis—a grotesque figure.

He was very tall, meagre, and yellow, with a long hooked nose, and small twinkling eyes. His head was cased in a woollen nightcap, over which he formed a flapped hat; he had a silk handkerchief about his neck, and his mouth was furnished with a short wooden pipe, from which he discharged wreathing clouds of smoke. He was wrapped in a kind of capot in green bays, lined with wolfskin, had a pair of monstrous boots, quilted on the inside with cotton, was almost covered with dirt, and rode a mule so low that his long legs hung dangling within six inches from the ground.

They crossed the Col de Tende, steps being cut in the ice for their frost-shod mules, by six hired men; near the top they climbed on foot, supported on each side by two of the men 'who walk upon snow with great firmness and security'. The descent was by 'sledge made of two pieces of wood', with one of the hired men in front 'with his feet paddling among the snow, in order to moderate the velocity of its descent', and another standing behind the sitting passenger. 'Thus accommodated, we descended the mountain with such rapidity, that in an hour we reached Limon', where most of the muleteers lived. 'Scarce a year passes in which some mules and their drivers do not perish by the valanches—balls of snow detached from the mountains which over-top the road.' From Coni they travelled by chaise on 'an open highway through a fine plain country, as far as the capital of Piedmont'—Turin. They took up their quarters at the Bona Fama, which stood 'at one corner of the great square, called La Piazza Castel'.

The doctor did not feel disposed to describe Turin and we do not know the length of his stay there. Presumably he returned to Nice by the same route as, if he had taken any other, he surely would have had something to tell us.*

HOMEWARD BOUND

The journey home began at the end of April and took them through Antibes, Toulon, and Marseilles, to Aix-en-Provence. The doctor had resolved to leave Nice 'without having the least dispute with any one native of the place' but, not surprisingly, he was not able to keep this resolution; he quarrelled with his landlord.

'The corn was in the ear; the cherries were almost ripe; and the figs had begun to blacken.' Antibes then lay on the frontier between France and Italy; Cannes was 'a neat village', a quieter, pleasanter place to reside than Nice—no walls or soldiers. For thirty miles they were distressed by the spectacle of the burned out pines of the Esterel hills; the work of some villains the previous summer. The local wine could not be nourishing as the peasants were so 'diminutive'; beer or milk would have been better for them. Wine, and all fermented liquors, were 'pernicious to the human constitution'.

Fréjus was a Roman colony favoured by Julius Caesar; its dilapidated amphitheatre was still being plundered of its stone by local monks building a monastery. Toulon was 'a considerable place . . . the quay, the jetties, the docks and magazines, are contrived and executed with precision, order, solidity, and magnificence'. Fourteen ships of the line were in its basin. Marseilles was a gay and flourishing city with an 'incredible' number of ships in its harbour. The long, semicircular quay was thirteen hundred paces in length, crowded with people and little shops. The galley-slaves worked in them, chained by one foot, and obliged to 'lie aboard' at night. But they looked well and jolly— 'shoe-makers, tailors, silversmiths, watch and clock-makers, barbers, stocking-weavers, jewellers, pattern-drawers, scriveners, booksellers, cutlers, and all manner of shopkeepers'. In the city there was a fine, wide, tree-lined promenade, a popular evening resort.

At Aix, the capital of Provence, once also a Roman colony, nothing remained of the temples, aqueducts and warm baths which had been erected around its springs. The doctor was told that the very source of the water had not been rediscovered until about 1704. At first it was only used for bathing sick animals; then poor people with skin disorders used

* Felsenstein doubts whether Smollett visited Turin at this time.

it. The physicians wrote about it and its fame spread. The waters were recommended for 'gout, gravel, scurvy, dropsy, palsy, indigestion, asthma and consumption' and many people at Aix drank as many as 'fourteen half pint glasses every morning, during the season, which is in the month of May'. Smollett took the treatment for eight days.

He touched up his narrative with a little 'science' here, saying that he did not have the proper means to make a 'complete analysis' of the water, but he understood that it did not produce 'agitation, cloud, or change of colour, when mixed with acids, alkalies, tincture of galls, syrup of violets, or solution of silver'. After bathing in it he thought his skin looked oilier, and when it was boiled, it gave off an odour of sulphur. The 'scorbutic' rash on the back of his right hand was 'almost cured'. But the winds from the north at Aix, made it unsuitable in spring or winter for people with pulmonary complaints.

The weather was pleasant as they travelled up the valley of the Rhone. There were no accidents or adventures 'worth notice'—only the usual 'abundance of little vexations'—'the Plagues of Posting'. There was a state monopoly so the traveller was at the mercy of landlords who were 'disobliging and rapacious', servants who were 'awkward, sluttish and slothful', and postilions who were 'lazy, lounging, greedy and impertinent'. Nevertheless, they had 'a continued song of nightingales from Aix to Fontainebleau'. At Avignon, the pope's title was 'precarious', and the noble bridge in ruins, but there was a fine city wall, and the tomb of Petrarch's Laura.

Orange had fine Roman remains, surprisingly well preserved. They stayed for three days at Lyon, which they reached on the seventh day out of Aix. At Beaune, they found 'nothing good but the wine'. At Chalons 'our axle-tree took fire'. At Auxerre they encountered another uncommunicative Englishman. He had broken an arm and Smollett sent him a message offering help. It was declined. 'This sort of reserve seems peculiar to the English disposition.' At Sens they visited a factory making 'Manchester velvet . . . under the direction of English workmen who have been seduced from their own country'. By the time they reached Fontainebleau, where they visited the castle, Smollett felt that his health was 'entirely restored'. But on the road to Paris they ran into a storm of sleet and hail, and he caught cold 'immediately'. It was 'reinforced' in Paris, where they lodged for three days. A night at Breteuil, another at Abbeville, and they were back in Boulogne, within sight of 'the white cliffs of Dover'. They rested there for some weeks before they felt bold enough 'to tempt that invidious straight' which separated them from England—a country he loved, 'because it is the land of liberty, cleanliness and convenience . . . and the habitation of my friends, for whose conversation, correspondence, and esteem, I wish alone to live'. It was June 1765 and he had been away for two years.

Published in the following year—1766—Smollett's *Travels*, not surprisingly, attracted criticism as well as praise. It was widely read, translated into German—but not in France*—and no doubt stirred up feelings of national pride and prejudice on both sides of the channel.

Laurence Sterne had been in the south of France at the time of Smollett's journey and had stayed at Montpellier. He too, at fifty, was suffering from chest trouble and tormented by 'scuffles with death'— and finishing the final volume of *Tristram Shandy*. Two years after the publication of Smollett's *Travels* he brought out his own *Sentimental journey through France and Italy*, dying a few weeks later in London. Sterne thought that 'the whole circle of travellers' could be reduced to the following heads—the idle, the inquisitive, the lying, the proud, the vain, and the splenetic. He called himself 'a sentimental traveller'—one 'who interests his heart in every thing, and who, having eyes to see what time and chance are perpetually holding out to him as he journeyeth on his way, misses nothing he can *fairly* lay his hand on'. Dr Smollett was 'Smelfungus'.

The learned Smelfungus travelled from Boulogne to Paris—from Paris to Rome—and so on—but he set out with spleen and jaundice, and every object he passed by was discoloured or distorted. He wrote an account of them, but 'twas nothing but the account of his miserable feelings'.

I'll tell it, cried Smelfungus, to the world. You had better tell it, said I, to your physician.

Another contemporary traveller, the eccentric Phillip Thicknesse, thought that Smollett's book should have been entitled 'Quarrels through France and Italy for the cure of a pulmonic disorder'. Dr Johnson, noting Thicknesse's words, told Boswell that 'There has been, of late, a strange turn in travellers to be displeased'.

English travel writers of the eighteenth century provided their public with many more books about Europe than about the British Isles, and it was the contrasts between protestant and catholic, the sober and the volatile, and the countries they inhabited, which was of such interest to their readers. There is a wonderful relish about Smollett's invective and his lines can still provoke that rare response—loud laughter. But prejudice and exaggeration and caricaturization, however popular and enjoyable, should be eschewed, said the Revd. J. C. Eustace in his

* Felsenstein says a French translation was printed in Geneva in 1792.

Classical Tour through Italy, 1802. Italy was no more peopled by 'dancers and buffoons, singers and fiddlers', and France with 'cooks and hairdressers', than England was with 'grooms and jockeys, cotton and woollen manufacturers'. And as for squalor and misery, Eustace said, there was more to be seen in our great manufacturing towns than anywhere in France or Italy. The Grand Tour writers, of course, did not describe such places.

But differences were looked for, remembered, and recorded. A picture would grow in the reader's mind, to which he himself might often be contributing. The streets of Genoa, to Smollett's reader, might seem full of people with 'the face of business'; to Dickens's reader they would have been 'all the better for the importation of a few priests of prepossessing appearance'. To both writers, the streets of Genoa were pleasing, and we can be sure that Smollett would have grinningly nodded his head on reading of Dickens's description of those monks and priests with 'repulsive countenances' who exhibited nothing but 'sloth, deceit and intellectual torpor'.

Smollett's health was not improved by his travels. 'I am returned to England', he wrote, 'after an absence of two years . . . I have brought back no more than the skeleton of what I was, but with proper care that skeleton may hang for some years together'. And it did so for another six years. He went to Scotland in 1766, and then to Bath. He still had the 'ulcer' on his right forearm. He thought he must have been 'in a kind of *Coma Vigil*' for some months of that year. 'I am now convinced that my brain was in some measure affected.' This was probably in reference to the weakness, lethargy, and melancholy he felt, and not to any cerebral pathology.

In 1767 he wrote to William Hunter that he was 'still crawling on the face of the Earth' and worried that his ulcer 'was become cancerous'. But he was still able to jokingly add that it was a 'Judgement of God' for 'the ridiculous use I had made of that wretched member in writing such a Heap of absurdities in the Course of my authorial Probation'.

He left England in 1769 and went to live in Italy, at first in Pisa. A year later he moved to Livorno (Leghorn). A villa on the slopes of Monte Nero was his final home. It was there, while he 'rusticated on the side of a mountain that overlooks the sea', that he completed *Humphry Clinker*, his most light-hearted and happiest creation. Hazlitt thought it was 'the most pleasant gossiping novel that was ever written'. In January 1771 he wrote to John Hunter;

With respect to myself, I have nothing to say, but that if I can prevail upon my wife to execute my last will, you shall receive my poor carcass in a box, after I am dead, to be placed among your rarities. I am already so dry and emaciated that I may pass for an Egyptian mummy, without any other preparation than some pitch and painted linen; unless you think I may deserve the denomination of a curiosity in my own character . . ..

But when he died, nine months later, his wife buried him in the English cemetery there. In 1974, his gravestone was still to be seen there amidst 'urns and sarcophagi, skulls and crossbones, broken pillars, cherubs, wreaths and medallions . . .'.*

For doctors, there is much of interest in the *Travels*. His ill-health was probably due to pulmonary tuberculosis, but what was the nature of the ulcer on the forearm? Not 'scorbutic', certainly. Some form of eczema? But there is no satisfactory description of it, in any case. And to what extent was Sterne correct, in attributing Smollett's jaundiced views and intolerant attitudes, to his complaints and anxieties? Few would be prepared to deny them a role but one feels that his own personality—forceful, extravagant, quarrelsome, and imaginative—had already been revealed in his novels. Novels in which travel, to the West Indies by *Roderick Random*, to Europe by *Peregrine Pickle*, and adventure were such a feature. And in *Humphry Clinker*, later, we are invited to participate in the journeys of a Welsh squire in the British Isles—an 'Expedition'—again described in the form of letters, in which Smollett displays his genius in observation and creative imagination in a truly brilliant manner. No character in his novels is more intriguing than the doctor himself.

But let us finish with some words from a Frenchman—E. Joliat, writing in 1935 in his book *Smollett et la France*. He reminds us that in the eighteenth century it was fashionable, in England, to ridicule the French; the English outlook was strongly Protestant and insular. ('Wogs begin at Calais' was the heading of a review of Felstenstein's edition of Smollett's *Travels*, in the Observer, 13 December, 1981.) In eighteenth century France, Joliat said, Smollett was highly regarded as a historian and writer; he was an accurate reporter and his novels were translated; but his sweeping generalizations were resented. Joliat quoted Tocnaye, a French refugee in England at the end of the eighteenth century. He had read Smollett and thought that 'If a stranger had said in England half of what Smollett had said in France, the people would have overturned his carriage and dragged him in the mud'.

Smollett in France was perhaps luckier than he deserved.

---

* *Paradise of Exiles; Tuscany and the British*, by Olive Hamilton, Andre Deutsch, London (1974).

BIBLIOGRAPHY

Anon. Tobias George Smollett. *The Practioner* **68**,195 (1902).

Anon. Tobias Smollett and William Hunter. *Br. Med.J.* ii,1096 (1904).

Beck, C. Tobias Smollett. *Am. J. Surg.* **32**, 383 (1936).

Brugsch, H. G. Tobias Smollett and Dr Antoine Fizès. A medical consultation in 1763. *New Engl. J. Med.* **254**, 383 (1957).

Dickens, C. *Pictures from Italy* (1844).

Drinker, Cecil K. Doctor Smollett. *Ann. Med. Hist.* **7**, 31 (1925).

Green, Robert M. Tobias Smollett: physician and novelist. *Boston Med. Surg. J.* **171**, 635 (1914).

Hamilton, Olive. *Paradise of exiles: Tuscany and the British.* Andre Deutsch, London (1974).

Kahrl, George M. *Tobias Smollett, Traveller–Novelist.* University of Chicago Press (1945).

Knapp, L. M. *Tobias Smollett: Doctor of men and manners*, Princeton University Press (1949).

Joliat, E. *Smollett et la France.* Thèse d. Paris, Honoré Champion (1935).

Jones, C. E. Essay on external use of water, by Tobias Smollett, M.D., edited with introduction and notes. *Bull. Inst. Hist. Med.* **3**, 31 (1935).

Jones C. E. Tobias Smollett (1721–1771); the doctor as man of letters. *J. Hist. Med.* **12**, 337 (1957).

Musher, Daniel M. The medical views of Dr. Tobias Smollett (1721–1771). *Bull. Hist. Med.* **41**, 455 (1967).

Noyes, E. S. *The letters of Tobias Smollett.* Harvard University Press (1926).

Smollett, Tobias. *Travels through France and Italy*, with introduction by T. Seccombe, Oxford University Press (1907); with introduction by O. Sitwell, Chiltern Press (1949); with introduction by James Morris, Centaur Press (1969); edited and annotated by Frank Felsenstein, Oxford University Press (1979); with an introduction by Christopher Hibbert, The Folio Society, London (1979).

Taylor W. D. Tobias Smollett, MD Aberdeen. *Aberdeen Univ. Rev.* **26**, 125 (1939).

Thicknesse, P. *Useful hints to those who make the tour of France* (1768).

Underwood, E. Ashworth. Medicine and science in the writings of Smollett. *Proc. R. Soc. Med.* **30**, 961 (1937).

6

John White's Voyage to New South Wales
1787–1788

JOHN WHITE served as a surgeon in the Royal Navy from 1778 to 1820. In 1787 he was appointed the Principal Surgeon to the 'First Fleet' to transport convicts to Botany Bay. It sailed under the command of Captain Arthur Phillip RN, who became the first governor of the colony of New South Wales. White's *Journal of a voyage to New South Wales* was published in 1790.

The decision to establish a colony in New South Wales by the settlement of convicts, was the outcome of several historical events and developments. During the eighteenth century there had been a slow realization in some quarters that the prisons of Britain were a national disgrace. But despite the humanitarian spirit which inspired individual efforts, there had been little legislative action and enforcement. A parliamentary enquiry in 1729 into the debtors prisons of Marshalsea and the Fleet, had been initiated by General Oglethorpe, a member of parliament. In 1733 he became the founder and first governor of the State of Georgia, the last of the thirteen English colonies in America. Georgia was intended to provide asylum to debtors and the impoverished of Britain, and to oppressed Protestants in Continental Europe, where the General had served for eight years.

With the loss of the American colonies in 1781, the unwanted could no longer be shipped across the Atlantic, and although some improvements had been made in British prisons, overcrowding and semi-starvation were still rife. In 1786, Lord Sydney, Secretary of State at the Home Office, recommending transportation, and no doubt mindful of the developing events in revolutionary France, said that 'The several gaols and places for the confinement of felons in this kingdom were in so crowded a state that the greatest danger is to be apprehended, not only from their escape, but from infectious distempers, which may hourly be expected to break out among them . . .'. South Africa had been deemed unsuitable, he said, but Botany Bay was 'a place likely to answer to the above purpose'.

Captain Cook, with the naturalist Joseph Banks aboard, had landed there in the *Endeavour* in 1770, giving the territory its name of New South Wales, and the bay where there was such a profusion of new trees, shrubs, and plants, that of Botany Bay. The sea, reported Cook, abounded in fish of all kinds, there were trees as tall and straight as pines, and others as hard as English oaks, and 'some of the finest meadows that were ever beheld'. Banks, by this time, Sir Joseph, President of the Royal Society and an influential friend of George III, recommended the site, and so Lord Sydney was commanded to signify to the Lords Commissioners of the Treasury his Majesty's pleasure 'that you do forthwith take such measures as may be necessary for providing a proper number of vessels for the conveyance of 750 convicts to Botany Bay, together with such provisions, necessaries, and implements for agriculture as may be necessary for their use after their arrival . . . '. This was in August 1786, but it was not until the following May that the fleet of eleven ships put to sea.

It comprised two warships, the *Sirius* and the *Supply*, six transports and three store ships, the majority being square-rigged with three masts. The transports were fitted out at Deptford, the convicts embarking at Woolwich, Portsmouth, and Plymouth. The fleet assembled at Portsmouth in March 1787 and when it set sail on 12 May there was 1500 persons on board, of which 759 were convicts; 568 males and 191 females, with 18 children. The ships carried a military force of 212 officers and marines, together with 28 wifes of marines with17 children. Although there were many hardened criminals and debauched prosti-tutes among the deportees, we should remember that transportation could follow conviction for many minor offences, such as larceny (over one shilling), poaching, stealing plants, roots of trees of the value of five shillings, setting fire to underwood, and, for Thames watermen, those who caused drowning of a passenger if a boat had been overloaded.

Surgeon White was worried about the lack of food and clothing provided at Portsmouth. Many convicts were in rags and had already spent four months in a prison ship on salt provisions. At Plymouth, 'A medical gentleman' informed him that there was 'a malignant disease of a most dangerous kind' among the convicts and that they should be 'immediately relanded'. White could not confirm this but found that the convicts kept to their 'beds' because of the piercing cold and their 'wretched clothing', their 'weakened habit and lowness of spirits' and the general effects of long imprisonment. He allowed the convicts on deck by day, 'one half at a time', and obtained promises of better clothing and improved rations. But the newspapers were full of alarming accounts of the distress of the convicts and 'letters from all quarters were pouring in upon us'. On one transport 16 men died before sailing. It is not difficult to imagine the chaotic scenes which resulted from the general overcrowding on the decks, where provisions, stores, casks of water, and pens for animals and fowl, restricted the movements of the crew, marines, and those convicts who were not manacled. The actual sailing was delayed overnight because of a protest about unpaid wages and final shore-leave on certain ships. White thought the trouble was caused 'more from intoxication than from nautical reasons' but it seems that pay had been witheld from many seamen by greedy ship masters.

White said that only one other merchant ship in the fleet had a surgeon. He sailed on the *Charlotte*, a three-masted two decker, 105 feet by 28 feet, of about 335 tonnage. She carried 88 male and 20 female convicts. The voyage to Botany Bay took eight months, which included a week at Teneriffe, and a month each at Rio de Janeiro and Capetown. They left Portsmouth on 12 May and arrived at Botany Bay on 20 January 1788.

West of the Scillies, after only a week at sea, two convicts were brought to the *Sirius* for a flogging as they were suspected of being the ring-leaders on one transport, having 'laid a plan for making themselves master of the ship'. Flogging is often mentioned by White, throughout the voyage; sentences of a dozen, two dozen, 100 and 200 lashes are listed. The first death occured on 28 May, one Ismael Coleman, who 'departed this life . . . worn out by lowness of spirits and debility, brought on by long and close confinement . . . he resigned his breath without a pang'. On 6 June, a second convict died, 'of a dropsy', having been tapped ten days before, with the removal of twelve quarts of fluid. At Teneriffe, which they reached on 3 June, a convict tried to escape by boarding a Dutch East Indiaman, but he was caught and punished.

At Teneriffe White accompanied Captain Phillip, and staff, to pay their respects to the Governor of the Canary Islands, and he visited Laguna, the capital of the island of Teneriffe. Two of the three hospitals there had been built 'for the wise, but ineffectual purpose of eradicating the *lues venera*', long common there. He thought that the natives resembled Pacific Islanders, but if he had been to the Pacific, it could not have been with Captain Cook. The latter left England on his last voyage, in 1776, two years before White enlisted.

They passed the Cape Verde Islands on 19 June but were unable to take on water and vegetables as planned, because of high surf, reefs, and haze. White said that many women suffered faints and convulsions from the heat, but the hatches could not be removed at night as the women invariably stole into the quarters of the seamen and marines for 'promiscuous intercourse'. The women were more troublesome than the men; their language and depravity apalled him. On some ships a few had to be put in irons or flogged, but punishment did not deter them. On 25 June, White visited the various transports and was generally pleased by the improved health of the convicts, but on 6 July, when 'porpoises passed through the fleet . . . like a pack of hounds scouring through watery grounds', Captain Phillip reduced the water ration to three pints a day per person. White was disturbed by this as he considered fresh water to be antiscorbutic. On a former voyage he had seen scurvy gums swell like a fungus and envelop the teeth, but subside in two weeks when milk and 'sour krout' were provided. On 18 July, rising bilge-water in one transport had blackened brass buttons and caused sickness. 'When the hatches were taken off, the stench was so powerful that it was scarcely possible to stand over them.' The bilge-water was pumped out, the water ration increased to three quarts a day and the 'sudden illness' subsided.

A seaman was lost overboard when he fell from a 'spanker boom' on one transport, and on another a female convict was fatally crushed by a boat which rolled from the booms. As they stood into the harbour of Rio de Janeiro on 5 August, Thomas Barret, a convict, and 'coiner', using brass buttons, buckles and pewter spoons, had managed to assemble 'excellent imitations' of the locally-used Brazilian silver dollars . 'The impression, milling, character, in a word, the whole was so intimately executed, that had their metal been a little better, the fraud, I am convinced, would have passed undetected'. A flogging followed, the seamen's grog issue stopped, the Brazilian authorities were warned, and one marine received 200 lashes for trying to smuggle one of the dollars ashore.

RIO DE JANEIRO

The month here was clearly enjoyable. 'It is one of the best harbours I have ever seen.' The wide bay and sandy beaches, the high surrounding mountains, the good wharfs and fine water aqueduct were all impressive—indeed 'romantic'. Officers were allowed to move freely, without escort, but unfortunately there were no inns or coffee-houses where they could spend the night ashore. There were some fine, long, straight streets, lined with three-storeyed houses; the ground floors were used as shops or quarters for servants or slaves. One street of shops was

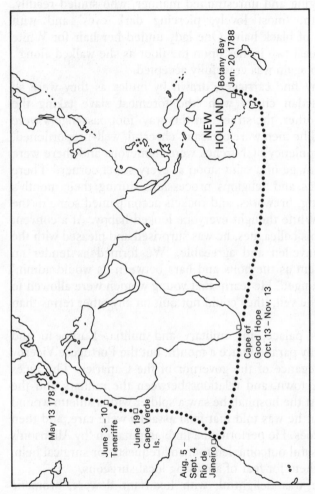

NEW
HOLLAND

Botany Bay
Jan. 20 1788

Cape of
Good Hope
Oct. 13 – Nov. 13

May 13 1787

June 3 – 10
Teneriffe

June 19
Cape Verde
Is.

Aug. 5 –
Sept. 4
Rio de
Janeiro

JOHN WHITE: VOYAGE TO NEW SOUTH WALES, 1787–8

almost wholly occupied by jewellers and lapidaries. White bought some topazes. Balconies and latticed windows were attractive features, and at some of them were ladies who 'by presents of nosegays and flowers . . . bestowed their favours'. In the street were to be seen 'unattended women', with engaging and unrestrained manner, who smiled readily, revealing fine teeth, 'most lovely, piercing dark eyes' and with 'prodigious lengths of black hair'. One lady untied her hair for White and 'it dragged at least two inches upon the floor as she walked along'. His offer to tie it up again was gracefully accepted.

There were many fine carriages, drawn by mules as they were so sure-footed, and sedan chairs with 'the foremost slave taking the pavement, and the other, the street'. In this way 'foot passengers were not incommoded'. The men were pleasant, cheerful, well-proportioned, 'but inclined to corpulency'. Churches were numerous and there were two convents. 'An image of a saint stood at every street corner.' There were several parades and religious processions during their month's stay; singing, dancing, fireworks, and rockets accompanied some of the secular occasions. White thought everyone looked happy. At a convent gate, with some of his colleagues, he was surprised and pleased with the nuns; they were unveiled and agreeable. 'We formed as tender an intercourse with them as the bolts and bars between us would admit.' Presents were exchanged. He learnt that young women were allowed to take a husband or the veil; 'they could not quit on any other terms than marriage'.

At the Viceroy's palace, the military and militia, European and Brazilian, customarily paraded once a month, but the Portugese Viceroy had none of the elegance of the governor of the Canaries. The races mixed freely in the town, and relations between the military and the public were good. At the hospital, he saw a soldier with a stiletto wound of the abdomen, but he was told that fatal assaults were rare, and then usually among negroes. He performed a limb amputation 'by Allenson's method'; the successful outcome led to many requests for surgical help. He had to decline them for fear of annoying local surgeons.

The countryside was delightful, with luxuriant flowers, aromatic shrubs, birds with colourful plumage, and 'an endless variety of insects with exquisite beauty and gaudy colours'. The cattle were small, but the beef was 'tolerably good'. Vegetables grew everywhere—cabbages, lettuce, parsley, leaks, white radishes, beans, peas, turnips, water melons, pumpkins, and pineapples. Then there were oranges, lemons, limes, plantains, bananas, yams, coconuts, and mangoes. He never saw 'finer flour for bread'.

On 3 September an English whaler bound for home, took their letters, and the following day the fleet set sail for the Cape of Good Hope, to a salute of guns from the shore battery. A convict received a dozen lashes for being insolent to an officer. This leg of their voyage took five weeks. There were favourable, but strong winds, and heavy seas. The convict ships rolled and pitched, one lost a fore-top-gallant yard, on another a convict fell overboard and was drowned. On White's ship, a convict, Mary Board, 'was delivered of a fine girl'. Sudden squalls and heavy rains caused some hatches to be battened down. What with seasickness and wet clothes, life below decks must have been miserable.

THE CAPE OF GOOD HOPE

On arrival here on 13 October 'The Commodore and Commissary went on shore and took lodings at the house of Mrs De Witt'. All were anxious 'to prepare themselves, by the comforts and refreshments to be enjoyed ashore, for the last and longest stage of their voyage'. Of course, as at Teneriffe and Rio, prisoners remained on board. There was some delay in obtaining stores and provisions from the Dutch; they said things were scarce, but in due course, fresh meat, vegetables and bread were purchased. 'The Commodore's sagacity and zeal for the service overcame the supineness' of the Dutch governor. They dined with the latter at his town residence and admired the gardens; they were 'as public as St. James's Park', handsome and pleasant, with well-shaded walks where 'many fashionable folk' strolled around, watched the birds, deer and ostriches, and a dozen or so wild animals on show.

Table Mountain, '1857 feet high', was climbed with some difficulty owing to heat and thirst. White tried chewing rushes and holding a pebble in his mouth. At the top—where a white cloud usually spread itself like a tablecloth in the summer season—they had a fine view of the town and harbour. There was a castle, several forts, twenty-three ships in the bay, and on the quay-sides, cranes and water pipes. The streets were tree-lined, but rough and unpaved. Roofs were thatched with rushes, not tiled, as they resisted gales better. A sure sign of an approaching gale was a rolling down of 'the white tablecloth' from the mountain. During their descent they spied some runaway negro slaves who lived on a high rock 'inaccessible to their owners'. They emerged at night to forage for food. 'The Dutch are not famed for their lenity in punishing crimes, but in general treated their slaves with great humanity and kindness'. During a three year stay in the West Indies, White said he had seen 'the infliction of the most brutal, cruel, and wanton punishments'. Dutchmen were large, stout and athletic looking; the ladies lively and good-natured, but very different in their habits from those delicate beauties on the romantic balconies of Rio. 'At the Cape, if you wish to be a favourite of the fair . . . you must *grapple* the lady, and paw her.' This 'rough approach' they found most pleasing. White caught a glimpse of some 'hottentots' (natives of the Cape); they were small, thin, dark brown, with woolly hair, thick lips, and daubed skins. They adorned themselves with ivory rings and strips of animal skin. He met a Dutch colonel who was writing a book about what he had learned of the hottentots and 'Caffres' (Kafirs, of the Bantu race) in expeditions into the interior. He admired the way the native drivers managed their teams of 14, 16, or 18 oxen, drawing heavy loads. These 'sooty charioteers', with a flick of their immensely long hide whips, controlled the oxen with effortless dexterity. Horse-drawn carriages were few, but there were many covered wagons drawn by three to six horses.

There were two churches, a large Calvinist, a small Lutheran. Near the Dutch East Indies Company garden, was a large hospital. At a parade of militia White was disappointed in the slovenly dress and unmilitary drill. They were a voluntary force, rather wild-looking, in long blue coats with white buttons. But his estimate of 'this burlesque on the profession of a soldier' brings to mind a similar underestimate when the British army faced Boer fighting men a century later.

On the day they sailed away, with livestock and fodder, a small American ship arrived, 'bound on a trading voyage to China with several passengers aboard'. They learned that a Dutch East Indiaman had been lost. A Kent whaler approached and also a Dutch ship carrying soldiers. They received letters from England via an East India packet.

FROM THE CAPE TO BOTANY BAY

This was the stage of the voyage which they most feared. It lasted nine weeks and there were many gales. The slower ships had difficulty in keeping up and scurvy and dysentery were ever threatening. On the first day out, Catherine Pryor, a convict, was 'delivered of a male child'. White visited one transport in which scurvy, attributed to 'damp and cold weather', had broken out among female convicts. On his own ship it was alleviated by 'essence of malt and some good wines'. A seaman was lost overboard, and another 'highly scorbutic' died a week after falling from a top-sail yard. A convict, Edward Thompson, died—'worn out with a melancholy and long confinement'. At times it was foggy and extremely cold; prisoners below hatches must have felt they would never tread again on land. And what awaited them in this new southern continent?

Food and fodder were in short supply; sheep died. But in spite of difficulties the ships covered long distances each day, up to 150 miles, when sails could be crowded on. Van Diemen's Land (Tasmania) was sighted on 5 January—'a bold irregular coast'—according to Captain Cook. A rock called Eddystone was sighted; named because of its resemblance to the lighthouse at Plymouth. At night they saw native fires. HMS *Supply* arrived in Botany Bay on 18 January, followed by three transports on the 19th, and the rest of the fleet on the 20th. They had travelled 15 000 miles. No one aboard had been there before.

'To see all the ships safe in their destined port', wrote White, 'and all the people in as good health as could be expected or hoped for, after so long a voyage, was a truly pleasing sight, and at which every heart must rejoice'. Two hundred years later, while admiring the mariners skill and courage, and the hardiness of all, it is the suffering entailed which stamps the stronger image on our minds. White recorded 48 deaths between embarkation and landing; 36 male and four female prisoners; and five of their children. One marine, one marine's wife, and one marine's child were also lost.

THE SETTLEMENT

White continued his journal for the next eleven months, until November 1788. When he concluded it, he explained that he had undertaken it at the suggestion of a naturalist friend, Thomas Wilson, of London. He sent home many preserved specimens of a botanical and zoological nature, and obviously spent much time observing and collecting in the new colony.

The fish were there alright, as mentioned by Captain Cook. They soon caught bream, mullet, large rays and 'smaller species', watched by natives who ran off into the bush when some officers ventured ashore. But it was an inhospitable-looking place. There was no spring water or grass to speak of, 'no fine meadows', and the bay itself was shallow and exposed. It was very hot, being high summer. Captain Phillip lost no time. On the 21st he sent the sloop *Supply* to investigate the entrance to the harbour a few miles to the north, which Cook had named Port Jackson. He had not explored it. On the 23rd the party returned 'full of praise on the extent and excellence of the harbour, as well as the superiority of the ground, water, and situation to that of Botany Bay, which I own, does not in my opinion, by any means merit the commendations bestowed upon it by the much lamented Cook and others'. Governor Phillip decided to start the settlement there, but as they were leaving Botany Bay, they were astonished and perturbed to see two ships approaching. But they turned out to be French vessels which had left France two and a half years before—on a voyage of exploration. They were looking for a beach where they could build boats and effect repairs, and they anchored in Botany Bay. There was an exchange of visits and the British fleet sailed off to Port Jackson on the 26th of January. White was delighted with it—'the finest and most extensive harbour in the universe—divided into a number of coves—Trincomalee is not to be compared with it'. In his *Journal* Captain Phillip said that he had

the satisfaction to find one of the finest harbours in the world, in which a thousand sail of the line might ride in perfect security. The different coves . . . were examined, and the preference was given to one which had the finest spring of water, and in which the ships can anchor so close to the shore that at a very small expence quays may be constructed at which the largest vessels may unload. This cove is about half a mile in length, and a quarter of a mile across at the entrance. In honour of Lord Sydney, the Governor distinguished it by the name of *Sydney Cove*.

On the 27th the landing of convicts, and remaining livestock (a few cows and bulls, horses, goats, pigs, fowl—and rabbits) was begun. Guards were mounted, lines drawn and patrols organized, and tents were erected. A start was made on a store house and the erection of the Governor's prefabricated house which had been brought from London. Sick tents were soon filled with cases of scurvy and dysentery. A vegetable plot was sown but the seeds blew away in the wind; the soil was hard. Plants withered, convicts went missing, five sheep were killed by lightning. On 7 February the Governor held a short ceremony and parade; the Union Jack was raised, volleys were fired and he addressed the troops and convicts. Criminal and admiralty courts were set up, and the Governor explained that he looked for obedience, industry, and honesty. 'He recommended marriage, assuring them that an indiscriminate and illegal intercourse would be punished with the greatest severity and rigour.'

The sexes had, of course, been separated for eight months and no doubt their re-union was noisy and dangerous. Nevertheless there were 14 marriages in the first two weeks.

A few convicts were found trying to join the two French ships. They were half-starved; one man and a woman were never seen again. Theft was common, everything had to be guarded. Punishments, as promised, were severe. James Barret (perhaps a relative of the coiner at Rio), a youth of 17, was the first to be hanged. He 'was launched into eternity' on 27 February for stealing some beef and peas. Next morning, two accomplices, 'about to ascend the ladder, were pardoned and banished'. Two days later, two more convicts had their sentence of death commuted to banishment. The latter usually meant a transfer to some barren rock or isle on bread and water for a stated time. On the 30th, a sentenced convict, with the rope around his neck, was offered a pardon if he undertook the duty of common executioner—'he reluctantly accepted'. An accomplice of his, in the theft of seven pounds of flour, received '300 lashes on his bare back with the cat-o-nine tails'.

There were two major difficulties soon encountered in the building of a settlement; lack of suitable timber and of limestone to manufacture cement. Most of the timber, White said, was fit only for firewood. None floated in water. There were many immensely large trees, 'clear of branches to an amazing height' and appearing to be ideal for shipmasts. 'But they were scarcely convertible to any use . . . at the heart, full of veins through which an amazing quantity of an astringent red gum issues'. There were other trees with 'a clear yellow gum'. They both went 'brittle' when cut and sawn, and 'fell to pieces'. These were the Australian Eucalyptus trees. Work was slow and laborious; 'I have known', White said, '12 men employed for five days in grubbing up a tree'. The men were of course weak from scurvy and malnourishment, and there was a lack of tools.

There was good stone, and very hard rock, but insufficient shells to take the place of limestone in the preparation of cement. White thought that oyster and cockle shells would be there in abundance. 'That great navigator [Cook], notwithstanding his usual accuracy and candour, was certainly too lavish in his praises.' At first they had to content themselves with 'cabbage-tree huts' and tents. In the fierce heat, on hard sun-baked soil, weak and ill-nourished men could not be expected to make much progress in the first months. Gangs of shackled men, led off into the bush to clear ground, under armed guard, was one way of attempting to start something—a prison perhaps, but not a colony. Some degree of freedom and imagination would surely have brought quicker results. Attempts to escape were inevitable; the majority died, were killed by natives, or recaptured. Violence, fighting, and thieving were countered with the severest punishments. Two men involved in assault were sentenced to 500 lashes each, 'but could not undergo the whole of that punishment, as, like most of the persons in the colony, they were much afflicted with scurvy'. A convict who stole a piece of soap worth eight pence was given 500 lashes. The hanging of two youths, one with post-traumatic amnesia who had been under White's care, 'made a great impression on the convicts'—as intended. 'They acknowledged the justice of their sentence . . . cautioned others . . . begged forgiveness . . . and prayed.' 'They were turned off; and in the agonising moments of separation of the soul from the body, seemed to embrace each other . . . .' We can only wonder whether such words truly reflected the doctor's thoughts.

If there was little imaginative leadership at the top, we can be sure that the convict who said he had discovered gold, was not the only talented rogue there. His specimens turned out to be 'a composition of brass and gold which he had filed down and melted'. He was whipped and branded. The governor did his best to explore the nearby countryside and to learn something about the natives. In April he went with a party to Manly Cove, for three days, 'so called from the manly conduct of the natives when the governor first visited it'. On a second expedition lasting seven days, White accompanied a party exploring the various inlets and trying to trace the source of a river. The ground was rocky and uninviting but White was delighted to see kingfishers, cockatoos, and parrots of various kinds. At night they lit fires to combat mosquitoes. They saw some canoes and came across trees in flame. They wondered whether this was the result of lightning, or the work of the natives, hollowing out trees to build bark canoes. Woods were sometimes impassable; they marked their path with hatchet cuts on trees—a practice 'called *blazing* in America'.

'The land', White said, 'the grass, the trees, the animals, the birds, and the fish, in their different species, approach by strong shades of similitude to each other. A certain likeness runs through the whole.' An observation which would have interested Charles Darwin.

'The singular anatomy of the kangaroo' fascinated him. Its immensely strong hind legs enabled it 'to bound along faster than a greyhound' and with 'its tail as a kind of counterpoise . . . and weapon, with which it thrashed a Newfoundland dog . . . while in its pouch was a young one not larger than a walnut, sticking to its teat'. A cassowary bird, seven feet high, with its long legs saw-toothed at the rear, but without a second stomach or gizzzard, was dissected. There was a remarkable structure of the feathers, with 'two quills with their webs arising out of one shaft'. The flesh tasted good 'not unlike young tender beef'. There was 'a vegetable tree', a shrub like 'wild spinage', 'a sage-like plant', and another 'with berries like white currant'. From a creeping vine they made 'a sweet tea' resembling 'the liquorice in the shops'.

The near naked aboriginees, 'without fixed abode', ventured to the shore from time to time, inquisitive but fearful. A soldier's uniform, or a musket, frightened them. They were amazed at the quantity of fish which could be caught 'while the seine was hauling' for they relied only on primitive spears 'pointed and barbed with the bones of fish and fastened with some kind of adhesive gum'. The settlers failed with the native spears; the natives stole the settlers fish. They carried shields of bark, stone hatchets, threatened and menaced men labouring in the woods, sometimes forcing them back to their camp or into the sea. 'They could throw spears ten or twelve feet long, thirty or forty yards with unerring precision.' White tended several men thus wounded; a few were murdered, others taken off and never found.

Two months passed before any big gathering of natives was encountered. On a beach, one day, 300 men, women, and children collected. The reason remained obscure. They grew less hostile as Captain Phillip approached them 'unarmed and with opened hands'. Gifts of looking glass, beads and fishhooks were offered. By signs the natives showed them what should not be eaten (toadstool), and what could (wood sorrel). White gave some uniform buttons to a girl who strung them round her waist, putting on 'a look of inexpressible archness'. Other females became 'coquettish' and some old ones adopted 'indecent attitudes'. On one occasion they saw two parties of natives assemble on a beach, select two champions, who then challenged, and fought with their spears. The women screamed when one was wounded. The natives would only eat meat if it was raw; they stole a puppy and ate it.

Things must have seemed desperate at times with food so short, livestock dwindling, and crops waiting to be raised. HMS *Supply* went off eastwards to Norfolk Island, a thousand miles away in the Pacific, half way to Fiji. It had been discovered by Cook. When the ship returned, at the end of March, it brought news of ample fish, a better climate, and of tall pine trees which could be used for building. On their return journey they discovered another island where there were large turtles and fowl. It was named after Lord Howe. In May there were many dead of the scurvy and the *Supply* returned a second time from Howe Island 'without a single turtle'. 'It was most alarming.' In October HMS *Sirius* set off to the Cape of Good Hope for wheat, and was not to return until the following May. It went via Cape Horn, thus circumnavigating the globe.

Three transports under charter to the East India Company left for China, in May 1788, eventually returning to England with cargoes of tea. In July, the three other transports, and one storeship, left for home, arriving there in the spring of 1789 after a journey in which scurvy decimated the crews and forced one of the ships to be scuttled. The birthday of King George III was celebrated on 4 June, with band music, parades, cheers and the singing of God Save the King; 'Every soldier receiving a pint of porter, every convict a half a pint of spirits made into grog'. A bonfire was lit. White was 'astonished at the number of thefts during the celebrations', and 'there was unabated depravity'. In August the temperature was low, the natives shivered on the beach and in their canoes; it was wet and 'the thermometer was frequently as low as freezing point'.

White ends his journal on a rather sad note, in mid-November, regretting their 'unsettled state', and appending a letter, dated 18 November 1788, from Sydney Cove, to Thomas Wilson Esq. of London. His book, with sixty-five engravings, of various specimens, many examined and dissected by the surgeon John Hunter, was published in 1790.

White's length of service in the colony is thus not recorded here but we know that Phillip remained as governor until December 1792, when he returned home because of ill health. He had seen the establishment of a settlement in the Parramatta river district, explored by the party White accompanied in April 1788, where the soil was better and where the first wheat crop was harvested in December 1789. It soon became more important agriculturally than the Sydney Cove settlement. Governor Phillip had a house built for him in Parramatta, in 1790, and nine years later, on the same site, his successor, Governor John Hunter, formerly captain of HMS *Sirius*, built a larger residence. This Old Government House, as it is called, may be seen today, fully restored, standing in Parramatta Park—the oldest public building in Australia.

Phillip also saw the arrival of the second fleet of convict ships in June 1790—bringing the first news from home and of the outbreak of the French Revolution. Dr White or his successor must have been sorely pressed to take care of the sick and dying, for the voyage had been a calamitous one, the result of overcrowding and wicked withholding of rations. There were 273 deaths among the 1038 convicts who had embarked, and 486 were ill. Phillip's report led to an outcry in Britain, the Colonial Office promised public inquiries, but there were no public prosecutions or convictions. The third fleet, fared better, arriving in July 1791.

Transportation of convicts to New South Wales continued until the eighteen-forties, and then, for a period in the fifties, to Tasmania (when the French were *starting* their penal settlement, on Devil's Island, French Guiana). It ended in 1868 in the Fremantle area in Western Australia. In eighty years nearly 170 000 convicts were transported.

BIBLIOGRAPHY

Bateson, Charles, *The Convict Ships 1787–1868*. Brown Son & Ferguson, Glasgow (1959).

Cook, James. *The journals of Captain James Cook on his voyages of discovery*, 2 Vols (ed. J. C. Beaglehole, Hakluyt Society). Cambridge University Press (1955, 1961).

Hunter, John. *An historical journal of the transactions at Port Jackson and Norfolk Island etc.* London (1793).

Lyte, Charles. *Sir Joseph Banks; 18th century explorer, botanist and entrepreneur.* David and Charles, London (1981).

Moorehead, Alan. *The fatal impact; an account of the invasion of the South Pacific 1767–1840.* Hamish Hamilton, London (1966).

Phillip, Arthur. *The voyage of Governor Phillip to Botany Bay; with an account of the establishment of the colonies of Port Jackson and Norfolk Island etc.* London (1789).

7

William Wittman's Travels in the Middle East: 1799–1802

WHEN William Wittman arrived in Constantinople in June 1799, his first impression was similar to that of John Bell sixty years earlier. Although he came by sea from the south—the best way—he, too, thought that the distant prospect of the city was the one to behold. The traveller, he said, should content himself with it for 'on nearer inspection he will find little to admire'. The Earl of Elgin had recently been appointed Envoy Extraordinary to the Sublime Porte, and Wittman had come as surgeon to the eighty-strong British military mission under General Koehler. This British presence in Turkey was in response to General Bonaparte's invasion of Egypt in July 1798.

Then only twenty-nine years of age, Bonaparte was already famous throughout Europe. Having saved the Republic in 1795, by 1797 he had conquered Italy and forced Austria to sue for peace. The Republic was already at peace with Spain, Holland, and Russia, and the British fleet had withdrawn from the Mediterranean. Only England and Portugal remained in the field against France. Realising that invasion of England had no chance of success, Bonaparte and Talleyrand turned their gaze to the east, aiming to strike at the power of England through Egypt and the land routes to Arabia and India. France had already proposed to the Porte that a canal could be built between Suez and the Mediterranean.

Sailing from Toulon, Marseille, and Genoa in May 1798, evading Nelson's newly arrived squadron, and taking Malta from the Order of the Knights on the way, Bonaparte landed his army of 55 000 from 400 ships, at Alexandria at the end of June. Within a month Cairo was in their hands, but on 1 August Nelson's fleet arrived at Aboukir bay and, destroying the French fleet, left Bonaparte and his army more or less isolated from Europe.

Egypt, then a relic of the Ottoman Empire, had been dominated by the Mamelukes for five centuries. By the mid-eighteenth century government from the Porte was only a matter of such things as appointing Turkish pashas in the various provinces of Egypt, collecting taxes and intriguing with the particular Mameluke beys in control of the citadel at Cairo. The fellahin toiled in the fields. During the autumn and winter of that year the French set up new administrations and laws, and chased the Mameluke horsemen up the Nile, to Karnak, Thebes, Luxor, and into Upper Egypt as far as Aswan and the first cataracts. Artists, archaeologists, and scientists of the Commission began their studies, the Institute of Egypt was founded, and in due course, in Paris, their collective scholarship was published in the two dozen volumes of the *Description de l'Egypte*—the only enduring achievement of the whole adventure. Other armies pursued the Mamelukes across the Delta into Sinai.

In December Plague broke out in Alexandria, Bonaparte's forces were being progressively reduced, no reinforcements could be expected, and the Porte declared war. For some time there had been rumours of impending invasion by Anglo-Turkish forces, by sea, or from Syria, and Bonaparte had to decide his next move. Dreams of conquering Constantinople and marching to India were entertained, but in February 1799, Bonaparte decided to attack Syria as a defensive move. Syria then comprised the present countries of Syria, Lebanon, Israel, and Jordan, divided into five Turkish provinces—Aleppo, Damascus, Tripoli, Acre, and Jerusalem. Bonaparte's campaign was almost wholly fought in what is now Israel. El Arish and Gaza were taken in February, Jaffa and Haifa in March. At Jaffa there was plague and the shameless massacre of Turkish prisoners. Acre, a walled city fortified by the Knights of the Crusades, was occupied by an Anglo-Turkish force. They were besieged by the French for two months before the latter decided to retreat. They marched back the way they came, suffering from lack of food, water, and decimated by dysentery, ophthalmia, and plague. They arrived back in Cairo in June after Bonaparte had lost about a third of the 13 000 men he had led on this disastrous invasion. But a month later he ably defeated a Turkish invasion army at Aboukir, and in August, promising to return, he slipped quietly away by sea with some of his generals and staff. Once again, he had the luck to evade British ships and land at Fréjus on October the ninth. He never saw Egypt again.

William Wittman arrived in Constantinople, then, when the French army was retreating from Syria. All we know of him from the Roll of Army Medical Officers was that in 1794 he was an assistant surgeon, and in 1797 a surgeon, Royal Artillery. After his tour of duty in the Middle East, there were further promotions, and in 1814 he became Assistant Surgeon General and Deputy Inspector of Hospitals, Ordnance

Department. He died in Paris in 1815; date of birth is not known. The title page of his book, *Travels in Turkey, Asia Minor, Syria, and across the desert into Egypt*, (1803), states that he had an MD and was a member of the Royal College of Surgeons of London. The book was dedicated to the Earl of Elgin, and among its 580 pages, there are many illustrations of poor artistic worth, usually of people and their dress and equipment. The test is straightforward, arranged in twenty-two chapters, and includes an appendix about mortalities, plague, ophthalmia, and climatic observations. It cannot be said to read with ease and enjoyment; though full of observation, the style is heavy, formal, serious. Indeed, in his preface he conceived it his duty to keep a journal 'in every respect consonant to truth'. He thought that 'Truth needs no ornament . . . what she borrows from the pencil is deformity'!

CONSTANTINOPLE

Wittman spent a year in the city, eventually sailing for Jaffa in June 1800. No European or Christian was allowed to reside in the city proper and he chose a house in the village of Buyükdere on the European side of the Bosphorus about twelve miles distant. It was delightfully situated, with fine views and pleasant walks, vineyards and orchards and wooden villas, and even a castle which reminded him of Dover. The countryside, he thought, may not have been the paradise which Lady Mary Wortley Montagu had depicted, but it was certainly enchanting. In his rides about the city and suburbs he soon became aware of the endemic diseases which had always characterized life around the Golden Horn. Blindness, lameness, and deformities were part of the street scenes, and there were always complaints of fever, malaise, dyspepsia, dysentery, and outbreaks of smallpox and plague. 'Herpetic and tettery eruptions' were common, but coughs were unusual. Three of the British staff died that summer, and one child was killed by a fall from a window.

He understood there were about 5000 doctors in practice—Turks, Greeks, Armenians, and Italians—all 'very ignorant'. 'Almost every individual in Turkey has a nostrum for some disease or other.' Elgin had his own child inoculated against smallpox and some Europeans followed his example, but few Turks were attracted to the idea, although Lady Montague had used it on her own children also, eighty years before, while in Constantinople. Variolation, as it came to be called, was replaced by Jenner's vaccination, which he reported in 1798. The old technique employed fluid from the lesions of smallpox; the new one, from cowpox. Rabies was there, too, and like Bell before him, and many

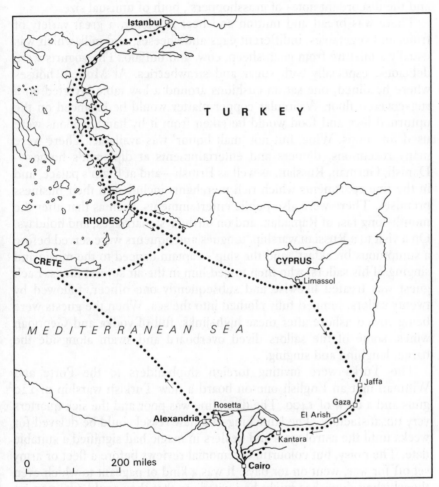

WILLIAM WITTMAN IN TURKEY AND THE EASTERN MEDITERRANEAN, 1799–1801

writers since, Wittman complained of the incredible number of half-starved, yelping dogs in the streets. Even in the suburbs there were new sounds; 'my ears were perpetually dinned by the croaking of frogs and the discordant notes of grasshoppers', both of unusual size.

There was bread and mutton and beef in plenty, a great variety of fruits and vegetables, indifferent eggs and cheeses, and milk which was usually a mixture from goat, sheep, cow, and buffalo. The yogurts were delicious, especially with sugar and strawberries. At Moslem houses where he dined, one sat on cushions around a low table inverted on a rug-covered floor. A circular copper platter would be balanced on the upturned legs and food would be taken from it by hand. Spoons were used for soups. Wine, but not 'malt liquor' was available. There were many receptions, dinners and entertainments at diplomat's homes— Danish, German, Russian, as well as British—and at Elgin's palace, and in the fine apartments which rich merchants included in their business premises. There were also public entertainments, such as that after the month-long fast of Ramadan, and on birthdays, marriages, and holidays. On a visit to a Russian warship 'tongues and liqueurs were served before a sumptuous breakfast', and the ship's captain danced to the music and singing of his sailors, who then tossed him in the air several times. Each guest was treated likewise and subsequently one officer, followed by twenty sailors, jumped fully clothed into the sea. When the guests were being rowed ashore after these high-jinks, full of vodka and Georgian wines, some of the sailors dived overboard and swam alongside the barge, laughing and singing.

The Turks were inviting foreign shipbuilders to the Porte and Wittman met an English one on board a new Turkish warship of 120 guns and a crew of 1400. The discipline was poor and the sick quarters very unsatisfactory. The launching of a new vessel could be delayed for weeks until the astrologers and dealers in magic had signified a suitable date. The noisy, but colourful ceremonial reviews before a fleet or army set off for war, went on for days. It was a kind of pageant to which even the whirling dervishes might be invited, so that they could summon up the spirits of valour. Wittman thought how strikingly it contrasted with the secrecy enjoining mobilization of a European army.

In general the Turks were grave, spending much time drinking coffee and smoking their long pipes. Greeks were gayer and nonchalant. Turkish women, rather short and corpulent, well covered up, were to be seen sitting around on grassy banks or tombstones, talking. Nails and hair were dyed with henna. Greek women were lively and attractive, with pale oval faces and black lustrous eyes, but they married early and aged rapidly. Greek men were not allowed to wear white turbans, only blue ones; neither could they wear yellow slippers or boots. Europeans, Greeks, Armenians, and other Christians had to pay all sorts of dues and taxes, and bribery and corruption were widespread. The great covered bazaar with its long crowded alleys and myriads of tiny shops, reminded Wittman, rather strangely, of 'our Exeter Exchange'. Special market police made daily rounds, checking weights and measures, and inflicting fines and punishments. A dishonest baker might have his ears cut off and nailed to his doorpost.

Robbers and murderers infested the city and roamed in large bands in the interior. When they ventured near the city a pasha would be sent off with an army to attack them. One returning pasha was invited to come to the gate of the Sultan's seraglio where he was saluted with praise and gifts, and then swiftly beheaded on the spot, because he had been suspected of corruption. After public executions the bodies were left hanging in the streets for days. On one day, 120 janissaries (Turkish infantry) and sailors were executed. When an army or navy was off to war, the streets were very unsafe, and people shut up their homes. A Turkish admiral was beheaded for allowing Bonaparte to escape from Egypt, and a rear-admiral only escaped with banishment to Cyprus for life, on the intervention of Elgin. A Turk who assaulted a member of the British mission was sentenced to death but Elgin succeeded in getting punishment reduced to fifty strokes of the bastinado and twenty years in a college in Pera 'to learn the Arabic language'. High-ranking officers were executed by the eunuchs, porters, or doorkeepers of the seraglio.

Wittman had a fever at Christmas and said that there were always rumours of plague; but there were actually deaths from it at Scutari at the time. He could not have felt cheerful. Corpses were buried naked and and not enclosed in a coffin. If death was due to the plague, the bier was covered with a red cloth. Wittman sent a pair of boots to be repaired at a cobblers, but plague was found in his house, the boots were not returned and the cobbler was sent off to a pest house. In February they learned that the plague was raging in Alexandria. During the winter, there were several deaths from the inhalation of 'mephitic vapours' from burning charcoal, used in braziers for indoor heating. Seven ladies in the harem of the Grand Vizier expired after suffering throbbing headache, nausea, and vertigo.

Wittman himself ended up with a throbbing headache after a visit to a Turkish bathhouse. He checked his pulse rate as he passed through the variably heated rooms. On a marble slab in the first, he was kneaded and manipulated; on a wooden platform over a hot stone floor, he was washed with warm water and rubbed with a glove of camel hair; lastly, he was lathered in soap, washed again, and enfolded in clean linen. Coffee and rest followed, with what benefit, he does not conjecture.

At a religious ceremony in a galleried, octagonal-shaped house, he spent an evening watching the whirling dervishes at their spinning-top, devotional exercise. He timed them as they whirled, first with their arms across their chests, then with them above their heads, and lastly with arms outstretched. Each man seemed to turn for twenty minutes to achieve 'a holy intoxication'. Greek celebrations at Easter were more enjoyable, with music, dancing, singing and wrestling in the streets and squares—'like an English country fair . . . with frying pans like a Bartholomew Fair'.

On a trip up the Bosphorus into the Black Sea he observed how the splendid old Byzantine fortifications had been neglected. The Turks, he said, knew that their empire was decaying but they were enormously suspicious and fatalistic, believing 'that they had received an assurance from the Koran that the empire would rise again in greater splendour than ever'. A Russian fleet was on its way to Naples; he met two Englishmen on one of the ships, one a surgeon in the Russian service. On another excursion he was away from Constantinople for five weeks. They sailed down the Sea of Marmora to Gallipoli, anchoring at the Dardanelles, where they were entertained aboard the flagship of the Kapitan Pasha, or High Admiral of the Turkish Fleet. The Pasha was originally a Georgian slave and had grown up with the Sultan, and remained a great favourite. He was elevated to his position purely as a token of friendship, having never served in the navy in his life. At the Dardanelles they were joined by Elgin and his suite, and they all went on horseback to the site of the ancient city of Sigaeum, on a hill overlooking the plain of Troy. They took away some marble, sculptured figures and inscribed bas-reliefs. They rode across the plain to Canakkale, a few miles north of the mound of Hissarlik where, seventy years later, Schliemann discovered the ancient city of Troy.

Throughout the winter and the spring, Turkish armies and fleets have been dispatched to Egypt and the British spent some time demonstrating the use of 'red hot shot', and other arts of war. Sick and wounded arrived from besieged Acre, but few from Jaffa. In January the British General Koehler and four of his staff went overland to Syria, returning, via Cyprus, in May. In February there arrived news of the El Arish Convention with the proposal that the French be allowed to leave Egypt, but it was never ratified, and the Turkish army suffered another defeat

by the French, near Alexandria. In April another Turkish fleet sailed off
for Egyptian waters.

JAFFA

The British mission sailed from Constantinople on 15 June 1800, into
the Aegean and down the coast of Turkey and the islands, to Patmos,
where they stayed the night of the twenty-first. Cos was another
overnight stop on the twenty-third, and, not delaying at Rhodes, they
sailed on to Limassol in Cyprus, arriving there on the twenty-seventh.
Leaving the next day, they reached Jaffa on 2 July, seventeen days after
leaving the Porte.

They were destined to spend the next eight months there, before they
marched off with the Grand Vizier's army to Egypt the following
February. It was a harassing experience. When Jaffa fell to Bonaparte in
March of the previous year, some 4000 people were massacred, most of
them Turkish soldiers. Wittman said 500 prisoners taken at El Arish
were also slaughtered at Jaffa. Then the plague descended and
hundreds more died. When Wittman arrived the scene distressed him.
The enormous encampment of the army of the Grand Vizier outside the
town, was dirty and disordered. There was little evidence of order and
cleanliness. Carcasses of horses, and camels and asses were strewn
about and, uncovered in shallow graves, were hundreds of human
bones. Fevers were rife, prickly heat was universal, jackals roamed the
camp, howling through the night, and thieves and deserters prowled
around.

'Dread and apprehension of the plague was everywhere', and in the
narrow streets of Jaffa blindness and malnutrition were only too evident.
Wittman judged that two-thirds of the population had lost the sight in
one or both eyes, speculating on the consequences of deficient diet and
local miasmas. Dysenteries and diseases of the skin were widespread.
Their own tents were moved to higher ground and a start was made on
clearing the site. As he rode through the olive and citrus groves he noted
the mud and straw huts of the impoverished fellahin and the dark tents
of the Bedouin—'all expert thieves'. In general, the soil was sandy but
there were fine acres of wheat, barley, corn, and cotton. The native diet
was based on bread, olives, cheese, and rice served as a pilau containing
portions of sheep or goat meat. Fish and fowl were there, too, but in the
whole of Syria he never saw a river.

The Grand Vizier's army was said to have had an effective fighting
force of 120 000—men of different hues, black, copper, olive, tawny,
yellow, and white—from Africa, Asia, Arabia, Syria, Greece, Armenia,

Albania, Georgia, and Tartary. The Tartars, as Bell had observed, were the most disciplined and amenable. The Turks were courageous and superstitious, ferocious and devout—praying five times daily. Turkish cavalry chose their own weapons—pikes, javelins, axes, or sabres, and a few muskets, carbines, and pistols. To the pommel of every saddle was strung a water bottle and a pipe. The camel drivers were Arabs; they had no tents and slept before the dung fires within a circle of their resting animals. The shaven-headed mercenaries from Morea, Macedonia and Bosnia—known as Arnauts—were the most formidable of the infantry. The Janissaries had been trained from childhood in the use of arms and were known to practise on prisoners of war and criminals. More important to them than their regimental colours, were two large copper kettles which were solemnly placed before their tents at night; there were two sets of them, if both were lost the regiment was disbanded.

Half of an army in the field would be composed of the camp-followers and tradesmen of every kind, coming from all quarters to bargain and sell. Wittman records how a couple of hundred camels disappeared with their drivers, the very night after they had been purchased. They were likely to be re-sold elsewhere. A lot of time and energy was spent in guarding provisions and livestock and pursuing thieves. The Pashas, of one, two or three horse-tails, and their commandants, weredecked out in distinctive robes according to rank and military or civil role. There were innumerable, traditional, but useless office-holders, with their special uniforms and accoutrements, such as 'principal and secondary dog-keepers' and 'bird keepers'. The most ridiculous of these over-costumed functionaries was the chief cook. He wore a garment of leather and metal, so heavy and cumbersome that he could not walk without the assistance of two lackeys. He was also one of those who wielded the instrument of punishment. No one of any rank moved about without an escort, each with their distinctive flags, standards, and banners. At night the thousands of tents were lit up by lanterns hanging from iron hoops on tall poles. There was no security and many a Turkish camp had been wiped out in a night. Desertion was common; one Albanian contingent of 500 sloped off after only a few days there, presumably learning of their poor pay and prospects.

The heat and dust and flies and diseases of the summer months must have been maddening. One wonders how he spent his time. He dissected some chameleons and located the cartilaginous ring at the back of the mouth where the flicking tongues were attached. He does not refer to sea-bathing or tell us whether he had any books. The present writer once spent a winter near Jaffa, during the last war;

bathing and riding were relished. He comments on the vineyards in the adjacent hills, but not on the wines at the monasteries he visited, although he refers to the *raki*, distilled from the fermented husks and stalks of grapes, and flavoured with aniseed. In the autumn, with General Koehler, his wife and several officers, he visited Jerusalem, travelling on horseback by way of Lydda, Ramle, and Latrun. They were met by the Turkish governor and Wittman stayed in a convent. They were conducted by monks on a tour of the holy places, and they went to Nazareth and Galilee. Wittman learned that when Bonaparte was in Nazareth he promised in the event of an attack on Jerusalem he would arrange that the first French grenadier to fall, would be buried in the Saviour's Tomb. A Mufti told Wittman that Jerusalem would not have been taken because there were '70 000 prophets' on the other side of the Dead Sea, ready to help.

Back at Jaffa, all seemed very disheartening. There was lack of water and provisions, sporadic shooting in the nights, thieves were bolder and desertions mounting. Many had had no pay for months and were feeling mutinous. In fact, a pay day was an occasion of pomp and ceremony. Bags of coins were displayed before the tents, and the High Treasurer with his attendants, resplendent in robes, appeared in procession, with pennants and music. For the Grand Vizier, there was more rumour than intelligence to be sifted. Arabs came from Egypt and the occasional British frigate brought news such as the recapture of Malta and the assasination of General Kleber, the French commander-in-chief, in Cairo. And from all quarters there was a ceaseless flow of rumour about outbreaks of plague. Pursuits and punishments went on. New levies from Acre arrived—without their noses, which had been cut off by the Pasha there. The governor of Damascus was beheaded after losing a battle with the French near Nablus. The Arnauts wielded their swords on the condemned. The severed head of a Moslem was placed under one of his arms, that of a European, between his legs, facing his body.

When the plague did descend, it soon raged. In December both General Koehler and his wife succumbed, as did thirty-six members of the Grand Vizier's family, as well as his chief physician. Soon, a hundred were dying each day, and at one field manoeuvre there were only 6000 troops. The British hospital tent was robbed. By the time they left, in February, many thousands had died. The Grand Vizier was saddened by all this, and Wittman, attending him one day, recorded that 'he laboured under great depression of spirits'.

The arrival of an English sloop with news of an approaching force from home was greeted with blessed relief. 'We were encouraged to hope that the painful situation of the mission would be speedily alleviated by the adoption of more active measures, which would bring the affairs of this part of the world to a speedy conclusion.' The mannered prose does not entirely stifle the *cri-de-coeur*.

THE MARCH FROM JAFFA TO CAIRO

For the frontispiece of his book, Wittman chose to illustrate 'The march of the Grand Vizier's army across the desert' which began on 25 February 1801 (Plate 18). Although a fighting force of 120 000 was probably an exaggeration (the majority of historians estimate one of 80 000) it must have presented an extraordinary, colourful, if noisy, disorderly, and malodorous spectacle. Mounted bandsmen led the initial parade, followed by the three horse-tails bearer, the pipe bearer, and the Grand Vizier with his Janissary and Mameluke officers. In the illustration we can see in the background a palanquin, cavalry, infantry, and a camel corps. There were wagons for provisions, water, and for the sick and wounded. Four months later, when they arrived before Cairo, they must have been a ragged horde, for lack of food and water, dysentery, ophthalmia, and the plague, had devastated their ranks. There was no effective supply organization and the march across the Egyptian desert, with insufficient tents, horses, and camels, became a nightmare, especially for the small British contingent.

They reached Gaza on 15 March and rested there for two weeks, Wittman noting the flowers, orchards, and tobacco fields. The houses were better than those in Jaffa and constructed of bricks of sun-baked mud with timbered roofs covered with thick layers of mud on which garden produce grew. The village had a green appearance, and but for a minaret, he said, might have escaped the eye of a passing traveller. Near the Egyptian border they learned of an Anglo-Turkish landing at Aboukir, and at El Arish on 30 March, they were relieved to hear that the plague was subsiding, and delighted to receive fruit and vegetables from Cyprus. The poor horses, however, had no barley for four days and were devouring their halters and dung; many camels died. Thirst, hunger, heat, and maddening khamsins led to abandonment of equipment and desertions. Leaving El Arish on 19 April they marched for seven days, in the early hours, to Kantara, where they found water and green grass, and managed to shoot some duck and pigeon. At Es Saliya, a few days later, Wittman estimated that they had crossed 150 miles of desert in 27 days. The temperature in his tent there was 112 °F. As they crossed the Nile Delta they saw their first mirages and were heartened by the sight of date palms and fields of clover and lentil.

Near Bilbeis, on 16 May, they encountered and threw back some French troops; 'the Grand Vizier had upwards of forty heads brought to him in the field of battle'. They were now more than twenty miles from Cairo, on the right bank of the Nile, and made contact with the Anglo-Turkish army which had defeated the French near Aboukir and forced them to retreat to Alexandria. British engineers had cut canals which inundated the region and surrounded the city with water. By the end of June Cairo was invested by the two armies and it surrendered without a shot being fired. The French left the city in July and in September they evacuated Alexandria.

The British Mission made their headquarters in the French Institute, which Bonaparte had set up for his scholars in a Bey's palace. During Wittman's eight-month stay in Cairo he found time to wander round the streets and squares, observing the clothes and customs of the people—Egyptians, Turks, Greeks, and Copts—the street touts with their charms and tricks and snakes, and the belly dancers. In public or private performances by the latter, he thought their motions were 'pliant and supple, rather than graceful', becoming 'indecent and animated' when the accompanying hautboys, flutes, tambourines and castinets mounted to a climax. Everyone was bare-footed and only Mamelukes and Turks were permitted to ride a horse in the city.

He visited the citadel, the mosques, the great aqueduct, the 'nilometer', a stone column which registered the level of the river, and the city wells, and he examined the obelisk at Heliopolis. At Giza he wondered at the three great pyramids and the sphinx. Some of his friends climbed to the top of the largest and into its burial galleries, but he contented himself with engraving his name near the entrance. He made some measurements of the head of the sphinx and said that the French had not found any animal body of proportionate size in the sand from which it protruded. He went up the Nile to the step-pyramids at Saqqara in the company of 'two gentlemen from Sussex'—Messrs Clarke and Cripps—who were on their travels. They returned to Cairo 'with a few vases and relics'. On another trip he went up the Nile to Helwan, near the first barrage. Processions of one kind or another were very frequent. Heading a marriage procession might be a henna-painted, decorated boy on a richly caparisoned horse; he was due for circumcision. He watched a caravan set out on its forty-day journey to Mecca, accompanied by 200 soldiers and 120 camels.

Plague was still about, even in their headquarters, but it was rife in Rosetta and Alexandria. A Dr White, who came with an army from India, did not believe it was contagious. Against Wittman's advice, he inoculated himself and his Arab servant, with pus from a bubo; he died four days later and his servant fled. In Jaffa, an elderly Scot named Campbell, who had been fifty years in the Middle East, a convert to Islam, and a General of Bombardiers in the Turkish forces, had also said the contagious nature of plague was a complicated question. It was not just a matter of physical contact, for resistance was influenced in mysterious ways. The master of a beautiful Circassian slave did not acquire the disease when she caught it, though he persisted to have intercourse with her, till she died. Isolation and quarantine were not practiced and when a plague victim was buried, the corpse was first washed and shaved. 'I am silent as the French', he said, 'on a theory of the plague'. He never mentioned rats or fleas.

In October, with two friends, he went down the Nile to Rosetta, Aboukir, and Alexandria. The Delta was inundated, villages drowned, fellahin and livestock crouched on elevations, huddling together, and only the water buffalos seemed contented. The planned inundation by the British was opposed by many because of the destruction it would cause. In some places he saw peasants at work in fields of flax, rice, and sugar, and on river banks there were indigo-makers. In the waters there were also floating bodies, human as well as animal. In Alexandria they saw Cleopatra's obelisk, the Pharos lighthouse and some mammoth-sized antiquities which the French had brought from Upper Egypt. The Rosetta stone, which a French officer had found in July 1799, Wittman did not mention, although the British General Hutchinson had succeeded in having it excluded from the loads of antiquities which the French were allowed to take back to France. And so it came to the British Museum. But it was a Frenchman who found it, noted the three types of inscription—Greek, hieroglyphics, and demotic—and had it sent to the institute at Cairo; and it was a Frenchman, Champollion, the Paris Egyptologist who finally deciphered the hieroglyphic and demotic inscriptions twenty-two years later, when he adopted the vital observations of Dr Thomas Young of London.

Wittman's duties at the Mission ended in February 1802 and he began the long journey home, going down the Nile to Rosetta, by sea from there to Alexandria (where he was quarantined in a lazaretto before permitted to enter the city), and embarking on a Greek corvette on 24 March. They had intended to land at Crete but storms drove them eastward and they were forced to seek overnight shelter on an island on the Turkish coast. They reached Rhodes on 8 April and enjoyed a stay there of eleven days. It was 'paradise'; no plague for six years and with a healthy, smiling population. Then, sailing northward through the islands, with halts at Cos, Chios (where there was a leper hospital, he visited), and Lesbos—all with their distinctive charms—they came to the Dardanelles, Gallipoli, the Sea of Marmora, and, on 21 May, Constantinople.

Anxious to get home to his wife and children, he embarked, two days later on a ship sailing to Varna, on the Bulgarian Black Sea coast. A week later he travelled north with a party of Greeks and Turks in a convoy of covered wagons. They were long and narrow, each pulled by one horse, and you could lie down in comfort. He hired three, one for himself, one for a servant, and one for his baggage. At Ruse, on the present Bulgarian-Roumanian border, he embarked on a Danube boat and sailed north to Galati where he met an English courier, a Mr Duff, who travelled with him across Moldavia via Iasi, into what is now the Ukraine, through Chernovtsky and Stanislav, into Poland. From Tarnow, to Cracow, and across what is now Slovakia, took them about a week in a horse-drawn carriage, arriving in Vienna on 19 June. During a ten-day stay there he heard the phrenologist Dr Franz Gall lecture on the brain and its functions—'broaching a new and dangerous doctrine'. He saw the splendid view of the surrounding countryside which the Austrian Emperor enjoyed from the apartment he had built on top of the circular-shaped asylum—*La Tour des Foux*.

With two officers on his Mission he went on by road through Linz, Regensburg, Nuremberg, Wurzburg, and Frankfurt to Cologne by 13 July. The last leg took them via Dusseldorf and Duisburg into Holland, and then to Arnhem, Utrecht, and Rotterdam by the seventeenth of July. Like so many English travellers of that time, Wittman exclaimed, no doubt with the squalor, pestilences, and corruption of the Middle-East still in mind—'I have not seen any country in which I could have resided with so much pleasure as Holland'. With what anticipation he must have embarked for Harwich, where he arrived on 21 July, 1802. And he piously admitted that he was grateful to have survived. Of 76 members of the Mission, 25 had died; of the 18 women and 16 children who went with them nine had died. And there were others, he learned, who had perished after he left Alexandria.

Heaven alone knows what the Mission had achieved.

BIBLIOGRAPHY

Denon, D. V. *Voyages dans la Basse et la Haute Egypte pendant les campagnes de Bonaparte en 1798 et 1799*, 2 Vols. London (1807).
Herold, J. Christopher. *Bonaparte in Egypt*. Hamish Hamilton, London (1963).

8

Henry Holland in Greece and Albania: 1812–1813

WRITING in his eighty-fourth year in *Recollections of Past Life*, Sir Henry Holland (1788–1873) said that over a period of fifty years, there were only two in which 'he had not passed two autumnal months in journey or voyage abroad'—and in those two exceptional years the autumns were spent in Ireland and Scotland. He was proud, even boastful, of two things—his travels and his circle of friends.

He made eight voyages to North America and Canada, four to the Middle East, three to Algeria, three to Russia, and several to Scandinavia, Spain, Portugal, Italy, and Dalmatia. He knew 'every single Capital of Europe' and many of the great rivers of the northern hemisphere.

The Danube I have followed with scarcely an interruption from its assumed sources at Donau-Eschingen to the Black Sea—the Rhine, from its infant stream in the Alps to the 'bifidus tractus' in Holland. The St. Lawrence I have pursued uninterruptedly for nearly two thousand miles of its lake and river course. The waters of the Upper Mississipi I have recently navigated for some hundred miles below the Falls of St. Anthony. The Ohio, Susquehanna, Potomac, and Connecticut rivers I have followed far towards their sources; and the Ottawa . . . for three hundred miles above Montreal. There has been pleasure to me in touching upon some single point of a river . . . as on the Nile at its time of highest inundation, in crossing the Volga when scarcely wider than the Thames at Oxford, and still more when near the sources of the streams that feed the Euphrates south of Trebizond.

Islands, too, had been on his itineraries—the Isles of the Aegean Archipelago and Levant, of the Canaries, Madeira, Caribbean, Gulf of Bothnia, Norway, Hebrides, Orkneys, Shetland, Faroes, and those of the English channel. Slight of figure, he enjoyed exceptionally good health, averring that in fifty years of practice 'he had never been prevented by illness from attending to the maladies of others'. He generally set out on his journeys alone, he could read and write in all circumstances, was never seasick, and his horsemanship was such that there was 'a flattering article in a Washington newspaper' about it, when he visited the Federal Army in Virginia in 1863. His energy was such, he said that 'On the day, or even hour, of reaching home from long and distant journeys, I have generally resumed my wonted professional work'. He recalled that there were patients in his waiting room when he returned 'from the mountains of Persia'. His first trip abroad was to Iceland in 1810, and his last, in 1873, to the north of Russia and the south of Italy (with a son). He died two days after arriving home in apparent good health, on his eighty-sixth birthday.

He also knew everyone. Even in his student days in Edinburgh he got to know Walter Scott, Lords Russell, Jeffrey and Murray, and when he settled in London he was soon friendly with Lords Landsdowne, Aberdeen, Holland (no relation), Byron, and Dudley, and Sir Samuel Romilly, Sir Humphry Davy and Madame de Stael; and in 1814 he was appointed physician to Princess Caroline of Wales, travelling in her party for a year on the Continent. In his *Recollections* he said he had known six British prime ministers and six American presidents, not to mention Talleyrand and Richelieu. When he was conferred DCL at Oxford in 1856, inevitably, it was in the company of such distinguished personages as the Crown Prince of Prussia, the Prince of Baden, Lords Clarendon, Elgin, and Lyons. After the ceremony Mr Gladstone said 'Pray, Sir Henry, may I ask what is your direction of travel this year?'

Holland was born in Knutsford, Cheshire, in 1788, the son of a medical practitioner. His maternal grandmother was a sister of Josiah Wedgwood, through whom he got to know the Darwins—Charles was 'a life-long friend'. Mrs Gaskell was a cousin who spent her childhood in Knutsford. He was educated privately in Newcastle and Bristol, where he met Richard Bright. After a few years as an articled clerk in a merchant house in Liverpool, he entered Edinburgh medical school in 1806, graduating MD in 1811. Bright was a fellow student there and they joined a five-month expedition to Iceland led by the geologist Sir George Mackenzie. The latter published a volume about it, *Travels in the island of Iceland during the summer of the year MDCCCX*, which included medical and biological contributions by Holland and Bright and some sketches by the latter. Mackenzie was pleased with them both and complimented them in his book, for their industry and cheerfulness.

In the Spring of 1812 Holland travelled to the Ionian Isles via Portugal, Gibraltar, Sardinia, and Sicily. From Zante he made two long, hard journeys through Greece and Albania. His journal, published in 1815, was entitled *Travels in the Ionian Isles, Albania, Thessaly, Macedonia etc during the years 1812 and 1813.* He settled in London and from 1820 till his death, his residence was 72 Lower Brook Street. His medical practice, he said, was 'limited very much to one district in London'. Success came early; FRS in 1816; FRCP in 1828; appointments to the Royal Household beginning in 1835, physician to the Queen in 1852, and a baronetcy in 1853. He is said to have declined nomination to the presidency of the Royal College of Physicians. An ardent member of the Royal Institution for many years, he was elected its president in 1865. Strangely, he was never on the staff of any hospital; he thought it would be too 'burdensome'. A *Lancet* obituary said 'nor was his face ever seen in public medical circles or at the Royal Medico-Chirurgical Society'. His practice was among the aristocracy; 'whether in actual medical attendance or not upon any sick celebrity, Sir Henry's carriage was to be seen waiting at the door, and he always had the latest bulletin of the patient's health'. But he early 'decided to keep my practice within £5000 a year'. He wrote essays about health, illness and medical practice, mental disorder and medical philosophy, in the *Quarterly* and *Edinburgh Reviews*, making no actual contributions to medical knowledge. As he said about his own practice—'it abounded, in truth, in cases which give little occasion for thought or solicitude, and are best relieved by a frequent half hour of genial conversation'.

He intended his travel book, of 550 pages, to be informative, and about those parts of Greece which were least generally known; he got to know the ruler of Albania—Ali Pasha—and described his character and rise to power. He provided a map and index, and included twelve engravings made from his own drawings.

THE FIRST JOURNEY

When Holland arrived in Zante in October 1812 the Ionian Isles were occupied by British and French forces. He recalled the long centuries of Venetian domination, the short Turkish rule towards the end of the eighteenth century, the French annexation in 1797, the 'Republic of the Seven Isles' of 1801, and the return of the French in 1807. Interestingly, he said that the French then 'aimed to restore various usages of the Ancient Greeks', including an Olympic Games every four years. 'These projects', he wrote, 'had a mighty aspect in the columns of the *Moniteur*, but that was all'. We can now recall that it was the French Baron Coubertin who initiated the modern revival of the Games, appropriately in Athens, in 1896.

The British invasion of 1809–10 resulted in Corfu and Paxo remaining in French hands, and Zante, Cephalonia, Ithaca, and Levkas, in British. The red face of the British soldier stood out among the swarthier countenances on the quay-side when Holland arrived at Zante, the British headquarters. He stayed there four days and found the people cordial and hospitable, despite their feuds and assassinations. British military families appeared happy, and their children were already speaking Italian. He remembered how Vesalius perished in a shipwreck there, in 1564.

In Cephalonia he learned that the profession of medicine was 'the favourite object of pursuit' among the quick-witted inhabitants. 'There is scarcely a large town in European Turkey where one or more Cephaloniotes may not be found in medical practice.' The majority were trained in Italy.

Taking a Greek guide he went north to Ithaca in an armed row-boat conveying money to the garrison there. Arriving at midnight, he wandered in the dark and empty streets looking for lodgings. Hearing the sound of billiard balls coming from a lighted house, he went in and soon found himself invited to stay at the house of one of the players, a young man of a well-known family. In his few days there, he met the Corsican governor, a fellow townsman of Napoleon, and a rather lonely couple—the British military surgeon and his wife. His host decided to accompany him to Yanina, by way of the island of Levkas, and Preveza on the mainland. They were a bit worried about pirates and were relieved to join the garrison at Levkas. This was the Leucadia of antiquity; there was a fine old Venetian aqueduct of 366 arches; houses were made of wood because of the history of earthquakes. Sailing from there into the Gulf of Arta, they saw the fortresses and new Seraglio, with painted walls and row upon row of small windows, erected by the Albanian, Ali Pasha. He had descended here with his warriors during the Franco-Turkish war in 1798. There was great slaughter and many Greek heads 'with their mustachios taken off', were sent to Constantinople, with the pretence that they were French. Holland recalled that in 31 BC, at Actium, a promontory opposite Preveza, was fought that great battle between the Romans and Mark Antony and Cleopatra. The ruins of Nicopolis, built on the north side of the strait by Augustus, after that victory, were visited—ruins of theatres, a stadium, a viaduct, walls, columns, and baths. The city had been razed by the Goths in the fourth century.

A three-hour boat trip from Preveza took them to place on the north shore of the gulf where they slept on straw mattresses in a noisy custom-house-cum-hostelry, where Albanians, smoked, drank and danced till a late hour. The next day, they tramped the ten miles to Arta, with a couple of horses to carry their baggage, over a road being constructed by hundreds of conscripted labourers, 'with a task-master standing over them with a lash in his hands'. On the rising road from Arta to Yanina they saw the semi-nomad shepherds with their great flocks of sheep—some two miles long—coming down from the snow-capped mountains of the Pindus. The men looked splendid and colourful in their small, round, red caps, bright vests and sashes, and woollen mantles reaching to the knees. They loped along on their rugged shoes turned up at the tip. The air was clear and exhilarating as they came up to Yanina, on the shore of a lake, with a striking back-drop of sheer mountain. On a peninsula reaching into the lake, and reflected in its waters, stood the fortress and seraglio of Ali Pasha, the Albanian despot from Tepelene who had established a virtually independent state in this part of the Ottoman Empire.

In the two weeks he spent in Yanina, Holland had several long audiences with Ali Pasha and he came to realize the formidable nature of his character. Yanina was a vital political link between Europe and Turkey. There were English, French, and Russian residents at his court, and he had agents in European cities and ports. Although Holland appreciated that Ali Pasha had cut a bloody swathe in his climb to power, he thought that one tyrant was better than many; he had united Albania and Thessaly, and Greeks were no longer in slavery. In the event, Ali Pasha was overthrown by the Turks in 1822.

Holland recalled the lines of Lord Byron, who had seen Ali Pasha in Tepelene, in *Childe Harold*

> Along that aged venerable face,
> The deeds that lurk beneath, and stain him with disgrace.

There were long medical consultations with Ali Pasha, but Holland would not disclose the complaints; he was invited to become his personal physician. He did not accept 'the gift of a girl', was not allowed in the harem, but saw two of the Vizier's 300 women. He heard that 16 of them were tossed into the lake while he was there.

The town had a population of twenty-five to fifty thousand, Greeks and Albanians. He stayed in the suburban house of a Greek merchant; in the city centre the majority of houses were made of mud. There were many bazaars, each with its own specialty—jewelry, shawls, groceries, tobacco, pipes, amber, leather, and pelisses. There were sixteen mosques, eight Greek churches, and two schools. Police patrolled the streets and no one was allowed out at night unless he carried a lamp or torch. Dogs were dangerous; two attacked him one day and tore his greatcoat. He saw eagles, kites, cormorants, and vultures, and ate fine fish from the lake. In a storm he saw a man struck fatally by lightning; there was a burn mark on his forehead 'where the electric fluid had entered'. As in some other modern regimes, emigration was controlled by preventing members of a family from joining a relative abroad. But he was impressed how Greeks managed to explore the commercial world; he met one family in which four brothers resided in four different cities—in Yanina, Constantinople, Moscow, and in Germany.

The passage across the mountains, on horseback, to Larissa in Thessaly, took six days; it was the usual route to Constantinople. A Tartar horseman could do that journey in six days and one was said to have been there and back in twelve. Two Englishmen joined Holland and Demetrius, and a Tartar was employed to look after the horses. The first night was spent in a khan; they supped on goats' milk, cheese, and wine. At Metsovon, perched 3000 feet up in the Pindus range, near one of the sources of the Arta river, they spent another night. The next day they travelled through the Pindus passage, or Metsovon Pass. 'It looked an impossible route', but the Tartar knew the way, and they reached the summit of the pass in two hours. It was a mere one yard wide; the temperature was 34 °F, the altitude 4 500 feet. Visibility was clear and they had a spectacular view down to the plain of Thessaly, and to Mt. Olympus on their left. Fleecy cloud hid the outline of the Archipelago which Holland, with accounts of Strabo, Pliny, and Livy in mind, hoped he would glimpse. Going down through the pine-covered slopes he estimated that during the day they must have seen some 400 horses on the pass. It was a busy commercial way. At Kalabaka some bandits had burned down a kahn and 'we had to trot hard for two hours'.

The rocks and monasteries of Meteora were extraordinary. The former rose to great heights from the valley floor in perpendicular masses and cones of conglomerate, with the monasteries, some dating from the thirteenth and fourteenth centuries, perched near or on their summits. There were originally 24, he was told, but now there were only ten. These 'aerial prisons . . . monuments of mingled vanity and superstition' were accessible only by ladders or in rope-suspended baskets hauled up by windlass from the top. Holland, with one of the Englishmen visited one of the monasteries—Aios Stephanos—climbing up a rocky path and then being hauled up in a basket, 150 feet. Demetrios used the ladders. There were five monks and a few attendants there; they saw the bare rooms, the simple chapel, and the library with its old books and manuscripts. In the refectory they were given rice, eggs, and wine for lunch. In this solitary hermitage he felt entirely separated from the world below—a mental state, no doubt, which the early abbots had in mind when they built them. (Patrick Leigh Fermor in *Roumeli*, 1966, describes this monastery of St. Stephen and the history of these 'Monasteries of the Air', and their present state.)

On the way down to the plain another night was spent at Trikkala where a local physician enquired about the teaching of the doctors, Cullen, Brown, and Erasmus Darwin, names 'known everywhere in Greece'. In a valley village they lunched on water-melons and quinces, the peasants greeting them with smiles; they had none of the rudeness of the Albanian. Crossing the river Pinios in 'a horse-boat', they soon had a view of the 24 minarets of Larissa in the distance. The Tartar went on ahead and two miles from the city they were met by a company of functionaries, soldiers, and physicians who escorted them to the house of the Archbishop of Larissa.

Dining there that evening, from a great pewter tray laden with soup, mutton, fowl, rice, and stewed pears, goat's milk cheese, and a dessert of grapes and olives, they learnt about Larissa. It was a mean, unattractive place, hot and dusty, liable to floods, 'with many negroes', and a population which was three-quarters Turkish. In their five days there, they thought the Turk an idle, unambitious fellow, 'his only movement that of raising or depressing his long pipe' and spending money only on his clothes. Met in the street, he looked dignified and well-dressed, but his home was always a wretched place. The industrious Greeks feared them and enquired whether England and France would help in their fight for independence. Holland said he met only one Turk who had any knowledge or interest in antiquity. The Archbishop felt anxious in the streets. Holland was impressed by the Sunday service in a Greek church.

Deaths from plague, that year in Constantinople, were said to have been about 30 000. In nearby Tirnavos, he learned that a physician from there, then practising in Vienna, had translated Oliver Goldsmith's *Grecian History*. There were several, lengthy, intermittent and tedious medical consultations for Holland. Three physicians would arrive with an account of the symptoms suffered by Veli Pasha, the son of Ali Pasha. Written translations would be made, a visit to the patient would follow—more waiting, more talking, more requests for written opinion and so on. The young doctor must have been glad to leave the place after five days.

With a new Tartar guide and a merry Dervish traveller with a mandolin, Holland set off north to Kattrini and Salonica. Mt. Ossa reminded him of Arthur's Seat in Edinburgh, and on its slopes, 600 feet up, overlooking the Pinios, stood the old town of Ambelakia, whose prosperity owed so much to the dye obtained from the madder root used in so many uniforms of the day. Along the narrow Valley of the Tempe leading to Mt. Olympus, he was again reminded of a place at home—this time, Bristol and St. Vincent's Rock. The cliffs were lofty, the pass five miles long, and at some points not more than 200 yards wide. It was difficult to imagine how Alexander managed to convey his army this way, from Thessaly to Macedonia.

They came to Kattrini, a town just north of the slopes of Mt. Olympus on 27 November; the nights were cold and and miserable in the villages through which they passed, but the Tartar seemed happy and warm, it was fascinating to watch him dress. There were two or three vests of embroidered purple velvet, three 'shawls' which he wrapped around his waist like a girdle, turning himself round and round in a dexterous fashion. With his silver-plated pistols, Holland thought his whole outfit must have been worth a hundred pounds. They sailed 'in a small bark' across the top end of the Gulf of Thermai to Salonica, a distance of twenty miles, taking eight hours. Built on the side of a hill, the city looked impressive from the sea, with its fortress of seven towers, lofty stone walls, domes, and minarets. There was a general air of splendour about the place. Its harbour was filled with shipping.

It was dark when they landed on 29 November and the gates of the city centre were closed, but they found a coffee house where they slept, with twenty other men in a large room; there were a few railed off, elevated areas and they secured one. The next day they met the English consul, a Mr Abbott, a merchant with a Greek wife, who had spent more than fifty years in various parts of the Turkish Empire, forty-two of them in Salonica. In the city there were few signs of ancient Greece or Rome; 50 per cent of the population was Turkish. There were three to four thousand Jewish families, mainly of Spanish descent, 'exhibiting the same active diligence here as elsewhere; but the repute of fraudulent habits goes along with that of industry'. A Salonica saying went 'Shun the Greek of Athens, the Turk of Negropont, and the Jew of Salonica'. Next to Constantinople, Salonica was the most important city in European Turkey and its commercial connections and routes were long established. By sea there were extensive trade exchanges, and by land there was a route through Bulgaria to Budapest and Vienna and Central Europe. Huge horse caravans were organized to transport corn, tobacco, and wool, and to return with grain and timber. There would be one, two or three hundred horses in a caravan—occasionally 1 000 horses. Each horse carried two packs of 1¼ cwt each. They travelled for eight hours each day, with one man to every five horses. At night there were armed guards and watch fires. The journey to Vienna usually took 35 days. One caravan set out during Holland's stay, which was worth £30 000 in Germany. With one of the Englishmen still with him, and the Tartar, they sailed from Salonica in a Greek brig on 5 December, heading down the Gulf of Thermai, for Stilis, at the head of the Gulf of Euboea. Normally a two-day voyage, it took them thirteen. They were driven eastwards by strong winds, and around the Northern Sporades, in sleet and snow. The Greek captain prayed to his saints in the cabin; they dragged their anchor near Skiathos, and, with dwindling food stocks, they sought shelter in an island inlet. Pirates were feared. A few wretched peasants gave them milk and cheese in exchange for bread. Arbutus berries with goat's milk and sugar formed 'an excellent dish'. On another isle they spent the night in a cave before fires. It was in these seas, said Holland, that Herodotus wrote of Xerxes losing 500 ships.

On the morning after landing at Stilis, Holland left the Englishman there, while he hurried up to Larissa to see Veli Pasha again. It was over the hills for about sixty miles; the countryside was poor and partly uncultivated; Holland had actually to stop his Tartar from whipping a peasant reluctant to sell them fowls. They reached Larissa in three days. Holland submitted 'a memoir in Italian' concerning Veli Pasha's symptoms; this was translated to the patient in Greek. There were more questions but he got away from the palace after two hours and was back in Stilis with the Englishman, and his Yanina Tartar, by 23 December.

They then turned south towards Delphi and Athens, where they arrived ten days later. Soon, their way narrowed between the mountains and the sea, and they came to the Pass of Thermopylae where, twenty-three centuries before, Leonidas and his Spartans had held up the army of Xerxes advancing upon Greece. Time had changed the scene; there was now no point 'where only a single chariot could get through'. In Livy's day the pass narrowed to sixty paces, now it was 300 feet in width and the sea lapped the road. Turning into the hills, the weather was cold and wet and they had difficulty in finding places to rest at night. In one village, near Salona, they slept around a fire in a mud dwelling with twenty other people and eight horses. 'Our bedding excited much surprise and admiration.' The peasants were frightened by the way Turks would commandeer a house; in one 'their beautiful daughter was smuggled away'. Holland was distressed by the way the faces of the peasants 'silently expressed an habitual expectation of ill-usage'. It was painful to contemplate and reminded him of the feelings described by Sterne in his *Sentimental Journey*. Just where Holland's party spent Christmas Day is not clear—but it could not have been a comfortable one. As they climbed through a pass in the Oeta mountains there were thick forests and deep ravines. On the descent to Amphissa the pathway was like a great, winding stone staircase, splendidly stratified. The horses stepped adroitly on the massive 'pavings'. The local commandant spoke English as he had spent some time in England on a mission for Ali Pasha; he had met King George IV.

To his readers, Holland explained that he was now entering the more classical districts of Greece, but that he did not wish to add to the familiar and well-known accounts of its ancient remains. At Delphi, in its solitary magnificence, the temples were gone—'where the splendour of art has disappeared, that of nature has remained'. There were fragments of marble and inscriptions scattered about and he saw 'the fine remains of a colossal statue which had been dug up a few days before, in front of a cottage'. Climbing some high cliffs above Delphi they turned eastwards towards Thebes, passing through Khaironia, Plutarch's birthplace, and Levadhia, where they felt three earthquake shocks and also enjoyed the hospitality of a Greek magistrate who possessed 'the most luxurious' home Holland had seen in Greece. It was fine and frosty on the Boeotian plain, with its fine fields of grain and rice and cotton, and ruins of old towns. But Thebes itself was a poor place, without any evidence of a classical past; its houses were chiefly made of mud, and there were a few bazaars and mosques. But the Boeotian women lived up to their reputation for beauty and were delightfully dressed, and decorated, with shining coins in their little caps or in the stresses of their long black hair. On the road to Athens there were more signs of classical history; remains, columns, inscriptions—and churches built from ancient marble. A night was spent in a poor dwelling belonging to a large family which was shared with two horses, nine oxen, two asses, beside their own party. But we must remember Holland was only twenty-four.

On entering Athens on 1 January, 1813, through one of its gates near the Temple of Theseus, one of the first persons they saw was 'an Englishman looking over an excavation', which prompted Holland to say that more than any other nation, it was the English who had 'cultivated the Ancients . . . thru Athens'. They spent a month in the city, Holland commenting that it was the wonderful combination of nature and art that made it so unique and uplifting. With the dry, arid climate, the extraordinary clarity of the light, the pastel shades of the classical monuments, and the grouping of the whole with their simple outlines—the Parthenon was unforgettable. Yet, although there was scarcely a house in Athens that did not possess some classical remnants, few Athenians were well-informed about their history. He enjoyed their company, being vivacious and hospitable, and the Turks, comprising about one-fifth of the population of 12 000, seemed to have lost some of their harshness. There were ten times more English, than French or German; most of the latter were artists employed by German courts. There was a great ball given to the European community by the Honourable Frederic North, recently back from a year spent in Syria and Egypt. The ladies 'were habited in the Greek fashion'.

In February they began to make their way to Corinth. The winter was severe and they met with much snow and sleet. The Tartar was replaced by a Janissary, a man of quiet nature but who proved of little assistance. They kept south of the hills via Eleusis and Megara, where Holland saw more inscriptions than anywhere, but they had to climb one mountain ridge through a guarded pass at 2500 feet. Corinth was a straggling place of 500 houses with a Turkish governor with his palace and fortress, a few mosques—and only seven pillars remaining from the Temple of Venus. Lord Elgin, in Constantinople, had secured permission for a visit by an antiquarian. At Mycenae, the rock citadel on the important path between the Gulfs of Argos and Corinth, the shortest route between Crete and central Greece, they inspected the impressive walls. There was the famous Lion Gate, the stone-paved roadway to the summit, the vaults and tombs and door to the Treasury of Atreus—where Schliemann was to make his important discoveries sixty years later. They reached the snow-bound town of Argus on 26 January where the thermometer read 29 ° F. From there to Tripolis they had a hard climb over the mountains. At 2000 feet they could see the island of Hydra, where, said Holland you would find the 'capitalists . . . the captains who became merchants'. For centuries they had been great traders in the Mediterranean; each voyage was carefully calculated financially—cabin boys having a share as well.

In the descent to Tripolis it was freezing hard; he attended a man who was in danger of losing a foot from frost-bite. There was 18 inches of snow in one village where they spent a night with a family of twelve, huddled around a fire. Slipping on the ice, they crossed a frozen stream on their horses and reached Tripolis. There they heard many lurid stories about the cruel Turkish governor of the Morea. A local physician who had studied in Padua possessed a much admired Voltaic pile which he used for the electrification of patients. Turning north again on 30 January—it was too freezing to go southward to Sparta, as Holland had desired—they crossed country not unlike the Highlands of Scotland. With a change of horses they reached Patras on the gulf, in three days, descending 1500 feet to the town. There, they met two Englishmen travelling to Zante, who had been delayed by pirates, but they managed to sail away on 4 February, reaching Zante that night. Holland had been travelling for three and a half months.

THE SECOND JOURNEY

This was a shorter one of two months in which he went north again by boat to Preveza, and through the Epirus to Yanina, and on to Tepelene in Albania. From there he went further to see the pitch mines at Selenice. Ali Pasha was at Preveza with his court and a few thousand soldiers, for the winter. They took him hunting by boat up the Gulf of Arta; Holland was disturbed by the way in which they shot at local fishermen. The Vizier supplied horses and an armed guard for the passage to Yanina. It was an arduous and at times dangerous ride; they had to negotiate rugged slopes, deep ravines and numerous river-crossings. Shepherd dogs were fierce and his clothing was torn on three occasions. At the fortress of Suli, the old commandant, who had fought with Ali Pasha, told him about their wars. From the gallery of the seraglio in which he stayed, one looked down into dark waters, amid scenes of wild, disorderly magnificence. The mountains and precipices around one, he found bewildering to the eye.

Further north, near the coast, one could see the French-held island of Corfu. At Paramithia, where some Greek bronzes had recently been found, an old Greek priest, merry on wine, persuaded Holland to look for ancient relics and treasure a few miles away. But they found nothing, and next day the priest confessed that he had been deceptive; 'but we concluded our acquaintance in good humour by making together a meal of eggs and goat's milk'. Again, in this area, Holland noticed how the Albanian soldiers would fire their guns at peasants working in the fields. They crossed a steep pass on the approach to Yanina, where, a few days previously, robbers had murdered a traveller. They spent the night in a guard house on the summit. An isolated amphitheatre in a valley surprised him. Known locally as Cassiopeia, Holland estimated it could have held 12 000 spectators. He had not seen Epidaurus but thought that it was not as large as this one. He took measurements but lost them later.

At Yanina he stayed a few days, seeing old friends and physicians, and then, with more armed guards and a passport, he went northwards through Zitsa to Delvinakion, near the modern Albanian border. Byron's description of the scenery was recalled; there were fine green hills and valleys, several hillside monasteries, and a splendid waterfall. The women were 'beautiful', and colourfully dressed. On the approach

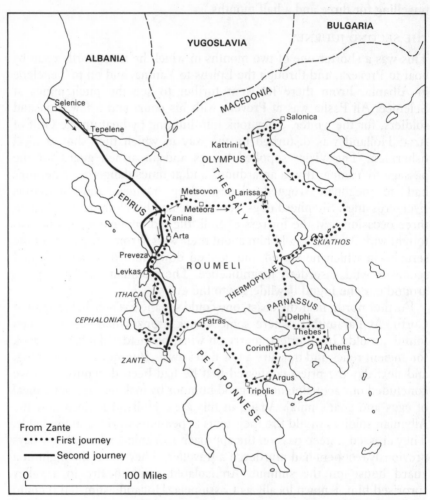

HENRY HOLLAND IN GREECE AND ALBANIA, 1812–13

On the map:

BULGARIA

YUGOSLAVIA

ALBANIA

MACEDONIA

Selenice

Tepelene

□ Salonica

Kattrini □

OLYMPUS

THESSALY

Metsovon □ Larissa

Meteora □

EPIRUS

Yanina

Arta

SKIATHOS

Preveza

ROUMELI

Levkas

THERMOPYLAE

ITHACA

PARNASSUS

CEPHALONIA

□ Delphi

Patras

Thebes □

Corinth

□ Athens

ZANTE

PELOPONNESE

Argus

Tripolis

From Zante
•••••• First journey
—— Second journey

0   100 Miles

to Gjirokaster, they had a splendid view from a mountain ridge; a long, broad valley, fertile with fields of corn, maize, rice and tobacco, said to be one of the most populated areas in Albania. Along one side of a river which flowed through it, he counted thirty terraces of vineyards, and through a gap in the hills one could look eastwards for twenty miles, to the town of Libohove.

At the seraglio in Gjirokaster, he saw the eleven-year-old son of Ali Pasha, who had planned the boy's education as a future ruler. After a year in Morocco when he was sixteen, he would spend five years in France, Germany, and Russia. His mother, in Tepelene, was rarely allowed to see him as 'she might weaken him by ill-timed indulgences'. The Moorish commandant in Tepelene was about ninety years of age; he had served in Ali Pasha's army and had a reputation for cruelty. Twenty years before he had roasted a man alive and a few days before, he had stabbed a man to death. His apartment was dirty and infested with cats and dogs, but Holland was given pleasant rooms in the palace and fine meals were sent in to him from the harem, by Ali Pasha's wife. There were twenty dishes to one meal. Holland did not see her. Employed in the palace garden was an Italian who had served in the French army in Spain. Captured by the English, he was eventually exchanged and joined the Corsican Rangers, and while serving in Corfu, he had deserted to the mainland and found work in Tepelene.

Inspecting an ancient site north of Tepelene, Holland lost his portmanteau on a ferry. It was probably stolen and he was greatly upset as it contained papers, journals and maps. He spent a day searching for it. At the pitch mines in Selenice he went down in a basket to see the tunnels where the black resinous substance was obtained. There were stories in classical times of fire emerging from the rocks and Holland amazed his guards when he lit gas bubbling from the ground; he trapped some in a glass jar. Each year, six or seven cargo boats loaded with 'asphaltum', left for Malta and the Italian coast.

On his return south Holland did not wish to spend more than a few days at Yanina, but Ali Pasha made him delay for two weeks; they had long talks each day and when Holland left he said that Ali Pasha actually rose from his cushions and kissed him on both cheeks. Holland was questioned closely about what he had seen in his travels and he suggested improvements which could be made at different places in Ali's kingdom. But the latter was primarily interested to discover if he had found any signs of gold and silver. Holland was provided with a carriage which took him to Arta, and he sailed back to Zante in mid-April 1813.

9

Richard Bright in Hungary: 1814–1815

In the autumn of 1814, Richard Bright, then twenty-five and recently graduated from Edinburgh, was travelling in Europe. He was the son of a Bristol merchant and banker and not yet settled in medical practice. He had been to a private school and had entered the University of Edinburgh in 1808, choosing not to serve a term of apprenticeship to a doctor. His studies were interrupted for five months when, as already mentioned, he and his student friend Henry Holland, joined an expedition to Iceland led by the geologist Sir George Mackenzie. In Mackenzie's book, Bright wrote on the botanical, geological, and zoological specimens which were collected, and Holland on some of the diseases encountered, among which were leprosy, scurvy, and infantile tetanus. They had taken a supply of anti-smallpox vaccine with them for the Danish doctors there, and had vaccinated some islanders. Bright also provided some sketches for the book—of a farmhouse, a church, a cliff cave, and a snow-covered volcanic peak which he had climbed. It was an arduous journey. The sea voyage from Leith, via the Orkneys, was a stormy one; a sailor was killed by a fall from the main-yard.

On his return, Bright chose to enter Guy's hospital in October 1810. He returned to Edinburgh two years later and graduated there in September 1813. Then, in the course of this unhurried preparation for a medical career, came a sojourn at Cambridge for two terms. Not deeming it a very useful place for him, Bright elected to set out for Europe.

After twenty years of war it was a devastated Continent which English travellers saw, that summer of 1814. With the abdication of Napoleon in April and his dispatch to Elba, they began to cross the channel again and to travel in a France forbidden them for eleven years. But Bright was bound for Berlin, through Belgium and Holland, and it was there that he heard news that sent him hurrying to Vienna.

The fall of Napoleon had left the disposition of his empire to the four powers who had overthrown him—Austria, Russia, Prussia, and Britain—and from all over Europe statesmen and delegates began to assemble in Vienna in September. There were hundreds of princely families, royal families with their retinues, and many thousands of visitors—the curious, the ambitious, and the inevitable hangers-on—writers and artists, actors and dancers, libertines and courtesans, thieves and street whores. The streets and inns were full, while in the palaces and assembly rooms, Talleyrand, Metternich, Castlereagh and their aides began that monumental carve-up of Europe, allegedly in the interests of 'common freedom and justice', which only restored the old pre-revolutionary dynasties—the Hohenzollerns, the Habsburgs, Bourbons, and German princes—to their ancestral domains. National aspirations were ignored; race, language, and cultures were not considered. Poles were shared by Prussia, Austria, and Russia; Norwegians were handed over to Sweden; the Belgians to the Dutch, the Venetians to the Austrians, and the whole of Italy retained its chequer-board pattern of small, foreign-dominated 'kingdoms'.

The news that Bright heard in Berlin was about this Congress. As it turned out, it was only one of the many rumours which periodically emanated from Vienna during that winter, reflecting the hitches and bargains and deadlocks which characterized the whole absurd business. 'I had already passed several months in Holland and different parts of Germany', he said, in the opening sentence of his book, 'when the expected dissolution of the Congress . . . induced me to hasten towards the capital; since I was naturally anxious to become a spectator of this most extraordinary assemblage'. In Dresden, a second message reached him that the Congress was over, so he stayed there for several weeks. Then, in Prague, he was told that a few days of it still remained, so he hurried on, arriving at the Danubian capital towards the end of November. He stayed there for three months and then made two tours in Hungary, before returning home in the summer of 1815, reaching Brussels just after the battle of Waterloo, where he saw the surgeons, some from Guy's, at work on the thousands of wounded soldiers.

VIENNA

This long journey led to the publication in 1818 of a large, handsome quarto volume of some 700 pages of text, tables and appendices, illustrated with engravings and woodcuts made from his own drawings. It was entitled *Travels from Vienna through Lower Hungary with some remarks on the state of Vienna during the Congress in the year 1814*. It begins with two chapters on Vienna.

He first lodged in 'a busy and dirty inn in the commercial part of the

RICHARD BRIGHT IN HUNGARY, 1815

From Vienna
•••••• First journey
▬▬▬ Second journey

0   30 Miles

USSR

ROMANIA

CZECHOSLOVAKIA

YUGOSLAVIA

AUSTRIA

Vienna
Laxenburg
W. Neustadt
Neunkirchen
Mürzzuschlag
Bruck
Craz
Furstenfeld
Eisenstadt
Sopron
Kőszeg
Szombathely
Körmend
Zalaber
Sumeg
Keszthely
Csurgo
Varazdin
Kaprivnica
Devecser
Vesprem
Varpalota
Székesfehérvár
Dunaföldvár
Szekszard
Pecs
Szigetvar
Budapest
Vác
Komaron
Gyor
Bratislava
Trnava
Urmeny
Nitra
Batha
Banska Stiavnica
Kremnica

Danube
Danube

city, which was much frequented by Greeks, Armenian and Eastern merchants'. His apartment was 'large and desolate, without a carpet, but provided with an earthen stove in one corner and a little wooden bedstead in another. Such are the miserable accommodations in most of the inns in Vienna.' The next morning, after breakfasting 'as usual in Germany, of a jug of hot scalded milk, and another of coffee', and after receiving a stream of visitors—barber, chiropodist, a couple of turbanned meerschaum pipe-salesmen, and a female toothbrush vendor—he sallied forth. It was a Sunday, the shops were closed, masses were being celebrated in the churches 'almost hourly', but the general scene was lively and the theatres opened in the evening. With 'a gentleman of Vienna' Bright went to a place of public amusement called the Redoute . . . where he was told he would have the opportunity . . . to see many of the distinguished persons then collected at the Congress'.

The Redoutensaal, as it is now usually called, is a great rococo-styled ballroom in the Hofburg. With its gilded ceiling and crystal chandeliers, its mirrors and Gobelin tapestries on the walls, it is a place where Mozart opera may still be heard.

We entered the room about nine-o-clock in the evening. It is a magnificent salon, finely lighted, surrounded by a gallery, and forming a part of the large pile of building called the Bourg or Imperial Palace. Never was an assembly less ceremonious. Everyone wore his hat; many, till the room became heated, their great coats; and no-one pretended to appear in evening dress, except a few Englishmen, who, from the habits of our country, and some little vanity, generally attempt to distinguish themselves by an attention to outward appearances. Around the circumference of the room were four or five rows of benches, occupied, for the most part, by well dressed females; while other parts presented a moving multitude, many of whom were in masks, or in dominos, and were busily engaged in talking and laughing, or dancing to the music of the powerful orchestra

Bright's companion took him by the arm and as they passed about the room, squeezing between gay groups of talkers, avoiding the dancers, and listening to the music, he identified many of the important personages who were present. Bright does not tell us who the Viennese gentleman actually was, but during the course of the night they were able to see in all their fine uniforms many of the notables from the courts of Vienna, St. Petersburg, Berlin, and Copenhagen, with German and Austrian princes and their followers. There was the Austrian Emperor himself, Franz I, 'a thin figure with shallow shrunken features, of mild expression, with a neck, stiff, bending a little forwards, and walking badly' (he was then forty-seven and lived another twenty years, so he may have had cervical spondylosis); the Czar Alexander I of Russia, 'his fine manly form, his round and smiling countenance, and his neat morning dress, were not to be mistaken' (Bright had seen him once before in a church in Haarlem, Holland; the Czar had been immensely popular with London crowds in June of that year); the King of Denmark 'a little man with white hair, a pale face, and aquiline nose'; the tall King Frederick William III of Prussia, with his 'solemn and grave features'; the King of Bavaria 'a large elderly man with a full face . . . like an Englishman'; the Grand Duke of Saxe Weimar 'a short thick old gentleman'; the Grand Duke of Baden, whose toes Bright trod on; the Crown Prince of Wirtemberg; the Crown Prince of Bavaria 'marked with the small-pox . . . speaking broken English'; the Duke of Saxe-Coburg 'stout and tall'; Prince William of Prussia, five Austrian Archdukes and Beauharnais (Napoleon's stepson), Viceroy of Italy, 'a fine dark military-looking man . . . with mustachoes'; and also an English milord wearing 'a remarkably flat cocked hat . . . two ladies in dominos leaned upon his arm'.

There were refreshments and suppers to be had in the adjacent rooms and galleries and 'the whole did not break up till a late hour in the morning'.

In this way for two or three hours, did we continue meeting and pushing amongst hundreds of men, each of whom, had he but made his appearance singly at a fashionabe rout in London, would have furnished a paragraph to our newspapers, prints to our shops, titles to our bazaars, distinctive appelations to every article of our address, and themes, if not ideas, to our poets.

'Such was my introduction', said the thrilled Bright, 'to some of the members of the congress'.

The scenes out of doors were no less attractive to Bright. In the Prater park the fine carriages and horses of the nobility and their friends presented a vivid and varied picture.

As the Emperor of Austria passes in one direction, driving the Empress in a phaeton with a pair of quiet horses, and a single servant standing behind, the Count Trautmannsdorf, the master of the horse is passing in the contrary direction, with a curricle or barouche and six. Immediately before the Emperor the carriage which impedes his progress is a fiacre, hired by a little shopkeeper to take his wife and child an airing in the Prater. Behind . . . are the impatient wheels of a tilbury, guided by a young English lord . . . next, a sort of truncated chariot . . . hired by a young Polish Count . . . the next carriage is an open landau, with four horses . . . it contains the King of Prussia and three of his diplomatic corps. Then the carriage of a wealthy banker; next a green *brishca* in which two young men are lounging at their ease; the cockade is Sardinian . . . now a carriage draws up . . . and the Pasha of Widdina lights with his companion, and followed by a man servant carrying his hookah, all are dressed in full Eastern costume . . . In short, the carriages and costumes of the whole of Europe, both civilised and uncivilised, were at this moment to be seen in the drive at Vienna.

There were aspects of dinner parties in Vienna which Bright thought 'of peculiar excellence'. An invitation to dinner, which was usually between 'twelve and five', did not necessarily mean that the guest would spend the evening with his hosts, or that the latter did not have an engagement immediately dinner was over. You might go for a drive, to the theatre or to some place of amusement.

The table is usually round or oval, so that each guest has means of intercourse with the whole party . . . it is covered, with a tasteful display of sweets or fruits . . . Each person is provided with a black bottle of light wine . . . the first dishes are always soups . . . [but] the succession of the dishes is not exactly the same as with us. An Englishman is somewhat suprised to see a joint of meat followed by fish, or a savoury dish usurp the place of one that was sweet . . . the conversation has been general and lively, and beyond a doubt, much more interesting than that which is heard on similar occasions and in similar society in England . . . both ladies and gentlemen rise at the same time . . . The party now adjourns to another apartment where coffee is served, and where it is frequently joined by other visitors. . . .

But the evening amusements at home Bright did not enjoy; they were often 'puerile'

Not content with requesting young ladies to recite verse, they will sometimes invert the natural order of things, and compel children to act plays, while the grown people play cross questions . . . .

Each chapter page of Bright's book is decorated with a vignette in the form of a woodcut depicting scenes he witnessed. 'A partial view of Vienna' decorates Chapter II in which we see the spire of St. Stephen's cathedral and the cupola of the Karlskirche, and we can catch a glimpse of the Glacis, the sloping green belt between the suburbs and the city, 'an intervening space entirely free from buildings'. Bright summarized the history of the city, the long threat from the Turks, the two sieges, and the humiliating defeat by Napoleon in 1805, when he married the Austrian Emperor's daughter, Marie-Louise, then eighteen, and took up residence in the Schönbrunn. The zoning and baroque expansion of Vienna which transformed it from a city-fortress in the eighteenth century, was brought to a halt during the Napoleonic wars. The modern city with its Ringstrasse, boulevards and stately buildings replaced the bastions and Glacis in the eighteen-seventies. At the time of the Congress, Bright said, the population of the city was about 270 000; a contemporary, and probably exaggerated claim was of the further influx of 100 000 visitors from all over Europe who had come to rendezvous in the capital.

Bright found 'a private lodging, and daily increased my acquaintance with the town and its inhabitants'. Walking in the narrow, paved streets and carriageways, was not very safe but coachmen usually gave warning of their approach 'by a species of unintelligible roar, a little in accent like the language in which a Lancashire carter converses with his team, but not less peremptory than the rapid "by your leave" of a Bath chairman'. There were the palaces and mansions to visit, the people and sideshows in the Prater, the public amusement park, and soirées, suppers, dances, and masked balls to attend. He seems to have had a busy and enjoyable sojourn.

'It was of course, one great object of the court to provide amusement for the strangers, and to afford the sovereigns as much variety as possible . . . [but] nothing of the kind could well surpass the magnificence of the species of entertainment, termed a Carrousel, performed by young men of noble birth . . . '.

The place appointed for this show was the Imperial Riding-School; a large saloon, surrounded by a narrow gallery about twelve feet from the ground, communicating with the apartments of the palace, and running behind the handsome Corinthian columns which supported a second gallery above. The whole was illuminated by chandeliers to a degree of brilliance which almost equalled the brightness of day . . . The seats at one end of the room were set apart for the Monarchs, and at the other for twenty-four ladies, whom we were to consider as the admired objects which would this evening call forth the utmost exertions of skill and prowess in the aspiring knights. At eight-o-clock, the heralds sounded their trumpets, announcing the entrance of these fair ladies, who, conducted by the champion knights, took their places of distinction. One would imagine that all the riches of Vienna had been collected to adorn the heads, necks, and persons of these four-and-twenty princesses. Their dresses of velvet and lace were covered with diamonds. They were divided into four companies, distinguished by the colours they wore;—of one party, the velvet was black, of another crimson, the third scarlet, and the fourth blue; and the mantle of each knight corresponded with the dress of his dame. The knights were in Spanish costume, splendidly adorned with gold and silver.

Bright went on to describe the entrance of the monarchs, princes, and potentates 'in their full uniforms, with their orders and decorations', forming 'the most magnificent assemblage of human beings which Europe could produce'. Twenty-four knights and their six-and thirty squires, all mounted on jet-black horses, entered the arena, made their obeisances and then, in groups of four, began to perform their feats of horsemanship and display. 'Figures had been placed in the arena, bearing the heads of Turks and Moors. Towards these each knight was to advance, and, passing at full speed, strike off in succession all the heads with his sword . . . .'

One Sunday, when the streets were covered in snow, the Emperor and his court, with the visiting royalty, paraded in a procession of sleighs to Schönbrunn. 'It was exceedingly beautiful.' There were some forty sleighs of various colours, 'adorned in the most splendid manner', with velvets and furs and ornamental gold and silver work. Each sleigh was drawn by a pair of horses, plumed and decorated, with fifty or a hundred bells around the shoulders of each horse, producing 'a lively and an agreeable jingling sound . . .'. Each sleigh carried a gentleman, and his lady, and was followed by a servant 'in a rich fur cloak'. He saw the torch-lit returning procession that evening and then 'I went to a little card party, and afterwards to one of the masked balls at the Redoute, where I laughed with great princes and flirted with masked ladies till a late hour'.

Music gets scarcely a mention. He refers to plays, theatres, and tableaus, and said that the Italian Opera was lately discontinued. But the only musical occasion he said he attended was at the Redoute salon when he heard 'a grand piece of music' by Beethoven, entitled 'Battle of Vitoria'. (It was at Vitoria, in Spain, that Wellington, in June 1813, defeated Napoleon's armies and practically freed Spain from French domination.) But there is no mention of Mozart's works, nor any other classical composer. Beethoven was living in Vienna, but his last public performance was said to have been about 1808. He died in 1827.

On the other hand, Bright was a good artist and linguist. He quoted Francis Bacon that 'He that travelleth into a country, before he hath some entrance into the language, goeth to school, and not to travel' (from his essay Of Travel, a much-used source of advice by young men on the Grand Tour in the seventeenth and eighteenth centuries). He found that the Poles and Russians were the best linguists. 'They acquire languages almost without trouble . . . on the contrary the English and French are most deficient.' Bright himself was clearly an industrious and vigilant traveller; his notes must have been voluminous.

Sunday in Vienna he found very different from 'our Sabbath rest'. He was there during Holy Week and wrote that 'The catholic festivals on the contrary appear to strengthen feelings which are always inclined to go beyond the reach of sober reason; they encourage people to indulge in the raptures of enthusiasm, instead of inducing them to enjoy and improve the solid advantages of domestic comfort and society'. That he was 'sober' and 'solid' himself the reader may judge from his prose; humour does not often break through. But then, he had warned in his Preface that the reader would not find in his book 'amusement derived from private anecdote', but rather, on the other hand, 'little more than the plain statement of the objects which were seen . . .'. To modern ears his style is often stilted and wordy, and at times quite fustian. Sometimes, when he allows himself, he writes in a lively fashion, and the pages are not so sombre. There must have been many tales he could have told, and conversations he could have recalled, but he soldiers on in an industrious manner, keeping to his prefatorial promise and eschewing such trifles.

We do, nevertheless, catch a glimpse of his nature from time to time. He was shocked by the way justice was administered in Hungary; the jails in the houses of the great estates, run by the nobility, he viewed with abhorrence. Another side of his nature is portrayed in the passage in which he describes, with open sentiment, seeing Napoleon's son by Marie-Louise, at the Schonbrunn. The child was then seven years of age;

. . . the sweetest child I ever beheld; his complexion light, with fine white silky hair falling curls upon his neck . . . He was dressed in the embroidered uniform of a hussar . . . continuing to arrange the dishes in his little kitchen . . . His appearance was so engaging, that I longed to take him in my arms.

This was the child called *l'aiglon*—the Duke of Reichstadt—who spent his entire life confined to the Schonbrunn (admittedly a prison of some 1500 rooms with a park of 500 acres, larger than Hyde Park), handsome and much-loved, dying there of tuberculosis when he was twenty-one. (His remains were removed by Hitler from the Capuchin vault of the Habsburgs after the fall of France in 1940, and taken to Paris; a crude attempt to bribe a country he had invaded.)

Bright's artistic temperament and knowledge are evident in the appreciative pages which he devotes to the various art collections in the city. Then, they were disposed in the various residences of the nobility, and represented centuries of acquisition and loot. Now, most of them may be seen in the Albertina and Kunshistorisches Museum, forming a rich, if ill-balanced, national collection. Durer's 159 drawings and engravings were of such 'delicacy and minuteness, combined with perfect freedom . . . when we remember the time in which he lived . . .', that Bright was tempted to consider 'the rich invention of his genius as supernatural'.

There were Rubens and Titians, Rembrandts and Vandykes, Murillos and Velasquezs to enjoy, and, as one would expect, hundreds of early German and Flemish masters. The collection of The Duke Albert of Saxe-Teschen 'would itself repay the visit to Vienna'; it contained 12 000 original drawings and 12 900 engravings. In the Imperial Palace there were vast collections of armoury, antiques, all sorts of *objets d'art*, and bronzes and tapestries. His days must have been very full. The Count Lambert's collection of 400 Etruscan vases obviously fascinated him. Listen to a few of his words about them which illustrate his zeal and powers of detailed observation. He is working out the Etruscan technique:

The whole of the process may be followed pretty clearly by observing attentively different vases. 1; The simply baked clay is seen, of a light red colour, on the bottoms of the vessels where there is neither glaze nor design, or where partial exfoliations have taken place. 2; Upon careful examination, indented outlines, traced in a rude manner, may be discerned, and sometimes lines of the same kind are seen even to intersect the figures. 3; Most of the designs are surrounded by a portion of the black paint, which, being higher than the general surface, has the appearance of a partial double coating, limited to about one tenth of an inch. 4; In one vase, found in an unfinished state, the black is but in part laid on, and looks like work done with a coarse hair pencil with paint not very fluid. I have some doubt, however, whether the first outline was traced after the first general coating, or whether it was not marked on the unburnt clay.

One feels sure that he would have delighted in the flowering of this Italian-born science of archaeology in the later years of the nineteenth century. He was disappointed by the lack of intellectual life in the city. 'The business of education in Austria is of a most formidable nature, both for its duration and formality . . . There is no philosophical or scientific community . . . government greatly discountenances all assemblies and societies of men, whether their purposes be friendship, scientific or political.' There was only one small medical society and 'a constantly superintending censorship' on all publications, whether foreign or indigenous. We may recall that Gall's lectures on craniology were forbidden in 1801 and he left for Paris. Even the words of Goethe and Schiller were only available 'in garbled and mutilated forms'.

It was a period of transition in the medical school and only Johann Peter Frank remained from the days of the Old Vienna School, of Van Swieten, Stoll, and de Haen. Auenbrugger, inventor of percussion in

1761, died in 1809, a year after J. N. Corvisart's French translation of the *Inventum Novum* had achieved fame for its author. Frank was in his seventies at the time of Bright's visit, but 'with all his faculties and dispositions . . . and with a great knowledge of books and men'. We remember him as the author of one of the first books on diseases of the spinal cord and for his great services to public health. Then, there was Hildenbrand, who bequeathed a classic description of typhus, and who, Bright said, did wards rounds with his students at seven in the morning, and lectured in Latin. He was impressed by De Carro who introduced Jennerian vaccination to Europe, beginning with his children who in 1799 were 'the first subjects of the cow-pox inoculation upon the continent of Europe'. There was Beer, who established the first eye hospital and published a well-known textbook of diseases of the eye. The chair of anatomy was held by Prochaska who is remembered by neurologists for his concept of a 'sensorium commune' and its part in 'reflection'. But his mercenary and secretive ways were disliked by Bright.

Prochaska is ready, for fifty ducats, to supply to the curious small cabinets, accompanied with a microscope, and containing about seventy microscopic sections, showing the most minute ramifications of different vessels in the various structures of the body.

Bright said that 'this art of subtle injection' had been lost after the death of Lieberkühn, and if lost again, it would be 'a blot upon the scientific spirit of the university of Vienna'. One is reminded of the secret material (wax, talcum, and cinnabar) which was used for the injection of vessels by Ruysch, the anatomy professor at Amsterdam, a hundred years before.

'The anatomical casts in wax, made by the skilful Florentine artists' which Bright admired, were undoubtedly those of Fontana, that extraordinary cleric, author of *The venom of the viper, The laws of irritability*, and creator of the museum of natural history in Florence. Anatomist, microscopist, and experimentalist, his wax figures can still be seen at the Josephenum in Vienna, and in Florence, Bologna, and Montpellier. The 'mannequin in wood' in the museum of the history of medicine in the Paris medical school, has recently been shown to be by him. Just as the Czar of Russia acquired one of Ruysch's collections for Leningrad, so did the Austrian Emperor Joseph II obtain a Fontana collection for Vienna.

'The magnificent general hospital', the Allgemeine Krankenhaus, built about 1783, around a series of open squares, was intended for

2000 patients, but had only 800 when Bright was there. 'The patients are distinguished into four separate classes, of which the three first comprise such as are not absolutely destitute, but are able to pay something towards the reestablishment of their health . . . cooks contract to furnish a full diet, a half diet, or a low diet . . . daily tested by some of the attending physicians in the kitchen and in the ward.' The wards were large, high and well-proportioned and heated by stoves; there were numerous small windows of 'double glass' which were never opened in winter. There was 'tolerable' roof ventilation, regular change and 'complete purification every six months'. There were eight resident physicians and surgeons. In the adjacent lying-in hospital there were arrangements for persons to be admitted 'in the most secret manner'; infants could be transferred to the foundlings hospital, if necessary. 'The moral tendency of such regulations may be a subject of animadversion; but their humanity is not to be doubted.'

It was in this lying-in hospital that Semmelweiss made his epic observations on puerperal fever in 1847.

'The asylum for the insane', known as *The Lunatics Tower*, 'is a fanciful edifice', thought Bright. It was a five-storeyed round tower, enclosing a square-shaped building, 'and not well contrived'. The circular building was for the 300 patients, and the other for staff. As at Bedlam and elsewhere the public were permitted to view the inmates as they would animals in a zoological garden.

As for the politicians and their Congress, Bright commented on the never-ending rumours and gossip, but 'I was never made privy to a single secret of these assembled cabinets . . .'. However, 'It was ever the anxious inquiry, whether England was the steady champion of justice . . .'.

Few writers about this historic summit meeting of 1815 fail to quote the *bon mot* of the witty Prince de Ligne, whose death during the congress Bright reported. It ran 'Le Congrès danse, mais il ne marche pas'. Bright, too, quoted it and we may suspect that the glitter he saw that winter in Vienna did not blind his judgement.

HUNGARY

That aristocratic institution—the Grand Tour—which was brought to an end by the Revolutionary Wars, had never included Hungary in its itinerary. It was the land-locked country of the Danube basin, between the Alps and the Carpathians. Roman invaders had been followed by Germanic tribes, and they in turn by the Huns (Buda was said to have been the name of a brother of Attila). The Hungarians, or Magyars, had arrived from the Urals in the ninth century. There was little of the classical tradition to be sought and savoured there by the aspiring tourist. It was still, in Bright's day, a feudal country. He sketched in its history and said that it was 'placed beyond the usual circuit of the traveller's observation'. But while in Vienna he had met some of the Hungarian nobility and they had provided him with letters of introduction. So, in March 1815, he said 'I embraced the earliest days of Spring' and set off eastwards with a friend along 'the road on the right bank of the Danube'.

He made two journeys into Hungary from Vienna, visiting Budapest during each of them. On the first trip he crossed the Danube into what is now Czechoslovakia at the town of Pressburg (Bratislava) and headed northeastwards by way of Tyrnau (Trnava) and Neutra (Nitra) towards the Carpathian mountains where he inspected gold and silver mines. He then turned southwards to Budapest, returning to Vienna via Raab (Gyor). During this journey he heard a rumour that Napoleon had escaped from Elba. In Vienna, when he learned that Napoleon had landed in Antibes and was marching with an army to Paris, he changed his plans. He had intended to visit Venice and Milan, and to return home via Paris. Instead, he re-entered Hungary, travelling southwards to Lake Balaton, and then to Varasdin in Croatia, now Yugoslavia. Turning eastwards he passed by way of Csurgo and Szigetvar to Funfkirchen (Pecs), and then northwards along the Danube, through Szexard (Szekszard) and Foldvar (Dunafoldvar) to Budapest. The return to Vienna took him through Styria and Gratz (Graz).

BUDAPEST

In 1815 there was only one bridge across the Danube linking the towns of Buda and Pesth (now there are eight).* It was 'a bridge formed of forty-seven large boats, united by chains and covered with planks', three hundred yards long and constructed so that sections could be removed for the passage of boats and rafts of timber. In winter the river froze over and the bridge was dismantled. On the heights of Buda were the historic fortress and arsenal, and around them clustered the palaces and houses, and the churches and theatres of the town. Pesth was the commercial centre; there were handsome houses, many erected around courtyards, and wide streets. The population of Budapest was then about 63 000.

* The suspension bridge built by the English engineer Adam Clark, completed in 1848, was the first permanent bridge over the Danube in Hungary. It was a duplicate of London's Hammersmith bridge.

Bright's drawing (Plate 25) illustrates the fine panoramic view obtained from the observatory on the right bank, with the wide loop of the river and the commanding position of the citadel.

He found an inn in Pesth which delighted him; 'a handsome new building [with] one hundred and ten bed-chambers, and an excellent coffee room on the ground floor . . . [providing]. . . tolerable music'. In the busy streets nearby there were peasants and dealers, ox-drawn rustic wagons and a variety of private carriages—fiacres and calashes. There were 'Jews, Armenians and Turks, each in the costume of their country', and at their shop doors sat merchants, usually 'between a bale of tobacco and a huge tub of caviare'. The baker 'trotted briskly from street to street' with a basket over his shoulder, 'announcing his approach by the shrill sound of a small wooden trumpet'.

Visiting the theatres he observed the different types of musical instruments in use. He sketched a *langspiel*, a stringed instrument which was plucked with a plectrum; there was the *dudelsack* or Hungarian bagpipe, and the *glockenspiel* or steel harmonica.

There were the warm public baths, some housed in ancient buildings of possible Roman or Turkish origin. In one he was overcome by disgust and heat; ' . . . it never happened before to me to meet, and, almost faint with heat, I was glad to make my escape'.

The apartment was spacious, the centre being occupied by a circular basin under a dome supported by pillars. The descent into this is by two steps ranging round the whole of its circumference. Here we beheld ten or twenty persons of each sex, partially covered by linen drawers and the long tresses which fell loosely from their heads, amusing themselves by splashing in the hot sulphurous water. Disgusting as this was, it formed the least disagreeable part of the scene. On the outside of the pillars, the floor was paved, and there lay, at full length, numerous human creatures, indulging, amidst the fumes, a kind of lethargic slumber; others lay upon the steps, and submitted to the kneading practised upon them by old women employed for the purpose; some, as if resting from their labours, lay stretched upon benches; and in the different corners were groups of naked families, enjoying their mid-day meal, sour crout and sausages, amidst all the luxury of a profuse perspiration. To complete the scene, there was a row of naked figures, like those in the bath, on whom a poor miserable surgeon was practicing the operations of cupping and scarification, studiously inflicting wounds, and making as much show of blood as possible, in order to satisfy the immoderate appetite of the Hungarian peasant for this species of medical treatment . . .

A far cry from the scene in the Pump Room at Bath, near his native city of Bristol.

In the university there were four faculties—philosophy, theology, law, and medicine—with six to seven hundred students, one hundred and twenty of whom were studying medicine. The course took five years and nearly all the lectures were delivered in Latin. A two-year course, in Hungarian, was also provided for 'surgeons who wish to practise in the country or small towns'. In the full course there was chemistry, natural history, anatomy, physiology, medicine, surgery, and midwifery. The small university hospital consisted of 'several small wards each containing six beds only'. Patients were grouped according to their sex and the nature of their illness—medical, surgical, diseases of the eye, and syphilis. 'Each [student] gives his report of the cases under his care in Latin; and on one devolves the duty of making a summary report of everything which has occurred in the course of each month.' Bright was 'much pleased with the order and regularity with which this hospital is conducted' and he thought that others could learn something from 'this distant and almost unknown medical school'.

As we would expect, Bright had to put up with much discomfort in his journeying through the country. He usually travelled in a horse-drawn wooden wagon or carriage such as that he sketched and used as a vignette (Plate 24). The roads were poor, sometimes 'there was literally no road', and often the carriage was axle-deep in mud. He said little about the details of his circumstances, what he ate, wore, drank, and so on. He tasted the wines, including the famed Tokay, found most of the inns 'miserable', and bed-linen unsatisfactory. In an inn at Weszprim, where he complained, he was told that 'very few persons had slept in the bed'. Such pests and nuisances as flies, bed bugs, cockroaches go unmentioned; there is no comment on drinking water or toilets. His complaints are not tedious or repetitive, like Smollett's, and he seems to have been tough and cheerful. That he was earnest and diligent is not in doubt. He had promised his readers 'information . . . respecting the state of the country', and this he provided. Geology, forestry, agriculture, industry, government, laws, constitution, towns, farms, estates, schools, churches and prisons, taxes and tolls are all duly considered, sometimes, in a rather wearisome fashion. Figures and tables abound. In an estate he will record the details of husbandry, and the rules and regulation, the listed produces, and the annual turnover. The reader will find pages on the cultivation of the silkworm, the keeping of bees, and statistics on the mines, the vineyards and arable lands. One feels that the dutiful son of the Bristol merchant and banker was 'doing his stuff' as it were, and anxious not to neglect anything which an English trader would wish to learn. On the other hand he is also informative about the different races and languages he encountered, and customs, dress, and behaviour are observed. He was sorry that he was not able to include a chapter on Hungarian literature.

THE PEOPLE

There were the peasants and the nobles; 'It is certan that the whole system is bad'. No one who was not a noble could own land; the peasant was 'bound' to an estate. As there was no strict primogeniture, estates tended to shrink, but a noble paid no 'tribute', 'tolls' or 'duties' and 'he goes freely through the country'. The wretched peasant, on the other hand, had 'scarcely any political rights' and was burdened with all sorts of dues and taxes, and was literally a 'slave'. A father of a peasant family owed 'one hundred and four days of labour during the year' to his *Graf*. One tenth of his products went to the church, and one ninth to the estate. Public works, such as the building and repair of roads and bridges, was another duty of the local peasantry. They also had to quarter and provision any soldiers and their horses who passed through. From garden rails in a village there hung 'a piece of board with two wooden hammers . . . employed as a drum to give the peasants notice to provide, at the appointed hour, provender and water for the horses'.

In his bedroom, at one estate, Bright saw a collection of notched sticks used to record the accounts between peasant and lord; the peasant possessed a duplicate, bringing it every other Sunday to be notched. 'All who are superior to the peasant look on him with contempt, mingled with suspicion and dread.'

The countryside generally presented 'no scene of rural delight'. There were few trees or hedges; a village might be no more than 'a wide muddy road', with 'two rows of cottages'. The peasants were usually unkempt but the Hungarians looked better than the Slovakians. The former were often colourfully dressed 'in hussar jackets, blue panta-loons, boots and broad-brimmed hats which gave them the appearance of banditti'. But the Slovakian peasant presented a miserable picture.

When you have seen one you have seen them all. From the same little head, covered with oil, falls the same matted long black hair, negligently plaited or tied in knots; and over the same dirty jacket and trousers, is wrapped on each a cloak of coarse woollen cloth, or sheepskin retaining its wool. Whether it be winter or summer, week-day or sabbath, the Sclavonian of this district never laids aside his cloak, or is seen but in heavy boots.

Many of these Slovakian peasants 'were afflicted by that unseemly disease known by the name of *Plica Polonica* [because of its appearance in Poland during the Mongol invasion of the thirteenth century] in which the hair grows so matted, that it is impossible to disentangle it, and becomes actually felted into balls, which, from an unfounded apprehension of bad consequences, the peasants are very unwilling to have removed . . .'.

Bright was surprised, therefore, by 'the appearance of comfort and good order' in many peasant homes. He depicted one in a sketch. There was a 'middle room or kitchen, with an oven constructed of clay' where bread was baked; a store-room which contained 'bags of grain, bladders of tallow, sausages and other articles of provision, in quantities which it would astonish us to find in an English cottage'. Bedding was stacked in piles and spread out on the floor at night. Between the houses were 'neglected yards and folds . . . and meagre cattle . . . and ragged children'. There were no gardens or flowers as a rule, and these Bright sadly missed. The village herdsman was a part of the scene. He drove the village herds of cattle, sheep, horses, and goats, 'a motley crew . . . better calculated to please the painter, than to gratify the skilful farmer . . .' out to the grass each morning, bringing them home at night. 'He carried a wooden trumpet, nearly four feet in length . . .' which he used to give notice of his approach. He was paid 'a small sum for each animal entrusted to his care, but part of this remuneration is always made in grain or bread'.

Rural markets were often enlivened by the appearance of peasants in their national costumes. There were Hungarians, Slovakians, Germans, Austrians, Wallachians, and Croations. In general, 'the female peasantry shew far greater value for their appearance than is usually found in our peasantry, except, indeed, in South Wales, where something of the kind is seen . . .'. He was told that by the 'way a handkerchief is tied around the face . . . you can tell the language they will speak'.

Then, there were the gypsies or *Cyganis*, to whom he devoted twenty-five pages. 'These people are spread through all Hungary, are distributed in every hamlet, but retain all the peculiarities which constitute a separate tribe . . . they seldom marry out of their body . . .'. They live on the outskirts of the villages, dirty and scantily clothed, usually occupied as smiths or carpenters, and carriers of messages and water. They helped in the fields at harvest times. They were forbidden to wear large cloaks, which could hide stolen goods, or own horses. He thought the gypsies were 'among the most curious phenomena in the history of man'. That after wandering around Europe for four centuries, acquiring languages, but not losing their own, Bright found astonishing. In some ways they resembled the Jews who also 'preserve themselves distinct amongst whom they are found'. The appearance, complexion and habits of life of the gypsies suggested an 'Oriental' origin. On his return to England he was intrigued to discover that some 'hedge-row' gypsies in Norwood were able to recognize many words he learned from the Hungarian gypsies.

Jews could often be recognized by their 'three-cornered hats, and cloaks like priests'. They were usually travelling merchants, 'buying at one town and selling at another'; he commented on 'the artful manoeuvres of these keen speculators'. Their immigration was con trolled and they had to pay a tax 'for the privilege of living in Hungary'.

The Germans received favourable comment. They were known for their 'superior industry', 'reliability', 'honesty'. The few examples of cottage gardens he saw belonged to them. In the vineyards, 'not content with procuring wine from the fresh grape, Ausbruch from the raisin, brandy from the skins, and syrup from the fermented juice, have likewise attempted to supply themselves with *oil* from the *stone*'. He was assured, at one place, when he was enquiring about the reliability of his transport, that all would be well, for 'the people are all German here'.

In one forest he was taken to see a settlement of Wallachians, a nomadic 'horde of one of the most singular nations which inhabit Europe, a nation ranking among the least civilised yet calling itself by the title of *Rumuny*' (Rumanian). They lived in huts of turf and wood, on the fringes of the forest, breeding cattle and sheep. They sat on the ground. The men were strong and many of the girls were handsome. He was told that in the Austrian dominions there were 1 600 000 of them; many eventually settling down in towns of mud and timber. They were harmless and honest, but the Hungarians were contemptuous of them. He made a sketch in the small settlement he visited.

CASTLES

On his first journey Bright stayed in a castle at Urmeny, north of the Danube, which is now in Czechoslovakia. Count Hunyadi was there for only one night, but Bright was accorded the warmest hospitality and every facility was placed at his disposal when he expressed his eagerness to learn about estate management. He was taken in hand by the 'Director', he met the family physician, the resident artist, relatives and children and in the next few days he learned much about the breeding of horses, sheep, and cattle. On a desk he found a copy of Tattersall's Racing Calendar; this delighted him for English experience had 'secured to Great Britain the finest horses in the world'. He examined the books of the estate and observed how everything, week by week throughout the four seasons, was counted, measured or weighed. He commented on the succession of crops, the yield of cows and buffalos, and the wonderful wool from the merino sheep. He visited many of the farms on the estate and enjoyed the views of the Carpathians to the north. But it was here also that he began to realize the drawbacks to this strange feudal system, and how neither landlord—nor peasant were content with their lot.

At Keszthely, at the western end of Lake Balaton, he stayed in the baroque-styled castle of Count Festetics, who had founded the *Georgicon* in 1797, the first agricultural college in Europe. There was a fine library of 15 000 volumes, schools of various kinds, and open-air music to be heard in the parks. Bright summarized the curriculum in a school for girls, entitled 'Objects of female industry'. It was a three-year course beginning with sewing and knitting and music, progressing to spinning, the care of silk-worms, and drawing and cooking. A modern visitor to Keszthely will find it a charming small town with a spa-like atmosphere, he can visit the castle and its Helikon library, listen to a concert in one of the parks, and at the main castle entrance he will find a plaque, unveiled in 1962, commemorating the visit of Dr Richard Bright in 1815.

At another castle in which he stayed, in Csaktornya, in Croatia, he referred to one of the unpleasant sights of the countryside. The feudal lord had the right of inflicting punishment on his peasants and 'in the very gateway of their hospitable mansions', prisoners in chains could be seen in the morning being marched off to the fields. The dungeons were 'dark and terrible recesses'; there were irons, chains, and flogging machines. The administration of justice in the local courts was 'barbarous'; the accused was not allowed to enter the court to hear the evidence against him, and the law officer had to conduct the case for both sides. Bright lamented the state of affairs.

MINES

Geology had been one of Bright's interests. He was attracted by the bleak and volcanic landscapes of Iceland, and lectured to the Geological Society in London, in 1811, on the strata in the neighbourhood of Bristol. In Czechoslovakia he visited the mines in Schemnitz (Banska-Stiavnica) and Kremnitz (Kremnica) and devoted a forty-page chapter to the mining of silver and gold there. The mining college of Schemnitz had been established during the reign of Maria Theresa in the seventeenth century. It lay 'in the bosom of a bold mountainous country

. . . the whose mass of mountain is a species of claystone porphyry . . .
[with] mountain caps of basaltic rock'. There were five principal veins,
each ten to twenty fathoms in depth, 'all connected at 200 fathoms by a
communication called the Emperor Francis's adit or level'. It was twelve
miles long.

Donning miner's cap, jacket and overalls, Bright went down by
ladders to 72 fathoms. It was cold, wet and noisy; a miner did an
eight-hour shift. The timber props were renewed every twenty years.
He studied the means by which water was pumped from the mines.
The machines, one of which he sketched, were themselves
water-driven . . . 'exerting its force to establish its equilibrium in an
inverted syphon, and acting upon a moveable piston by its hydrostatic
pressure'. He described the work entailed in raising the ores, washing
and preparing them, and in the smelting, refining, and extraction of gold
and silver. He visited the Royal Mints where the ingots were made and
stamped. German was the language used and he found the Hohenhaus
'one of the best inns I had encountered on the Continent'.

He was accordingly surprised to learn that 'an officer, connected with
the most celebrated source of gold and silver in Europe, should still
believe that Mexico is an English island and that other clever and
agreeable persons could scarcely be convinced that coffee, and sugar,
and rice, are not products of Great Britain'.

On leaving the mines, one of the inspectors 'saluted me on both
cheeks; a compliment frequent on the Continent, but which an
Englishman can with difficulty bring himself to return'.

Turning towards home after his second journey we sense a degree of
maladie du pays when, in an estate, he 'fancied himself in England' at the
sight of some flower gardens. It was of a style 'universally called on the
Continent *English*, that is, a style in which art is not allowed to disguise
nature'. He had been happy in Hungary and wished their people well.
The country was placed in 'a commanding situation as the portal and
barrier of the east' and he hoped that 'free and powerful nobles will be
the lords of a free and powerful peasantry'. But England called.

We are not always sufficiently aware how great an influence is excited by trifling
circumstances in the formation of important traits of national character. I am
strongly inclined to believe that the blazing hearth and the comfortable carpet
do more to form the domestic character of the English nation, than any original
disposition or physical temperament; and that the crowded theatres and
tea-gardens of the Continent give evidence of the want of comfort at home,
rather than of the gaiety of the heart. Were I the proprietor of an Hungarian
estate, my first attempt would be, to encourage my peasantry to cultivate their

flower-gardens, certain as I should feel, that, by this means, I was strengthening their attachment to their homes, to the country, and to their hereditary lord; and I should never be better satisfied, than when every ploughman, and every shepherdess on my estate, could present my children with a finer nosegay than my own garden could produce—when the village church should be filled with the fresh incense of the rose and the violet, and every grave be strewed with their blossoms.

The year or so Bright spent in Europe probably influenced his outlook in many ways as well as sharpening his powers of observation. But those traits of character by which he generally came to be appreciated, may be readily discerned in his travel book. From the *Dictionary of National Biography* we learn that he possessed 'an affectionate disposition', was 'uniformly cheerful', and that 'his industry was indefatigable'. Dr Wilks wrote that 'we are struck with astonishment at his powers of observation'. Bright 'was not generally regarded as a brilliant man' and 'he had little powers of exposition'. He did not theorise and there was 'a certain simplicity in his intellectual character'. In Munk's Roll of the Royal College of Physicians of London, we read that 'he was sincerely religious both in doctrine and practice and of so pure a mind that he never was heard to utter a sentiment or to relate an anecdote that was not fit to be heard by the merest child or the most refined female . . .'. So we can rest assured that those beautiful girls in the forest and those masked ladies in Vienna would have had a difficult time in trying to seduce him.

Bright's book received a twenty-two page review in the *Edinburgh Review* of 1818 (Vol. 31, p. 214). The anonymous writer said 'This is evidently the work of a very amiable and intelligent man, who has observed, with the utmost diligence, everything remarkable that came within the sphere of his observations, and set down in his book, perhaps with too much minuteness, everything that he had so observed'. The narrative was lively and pleasant and there was cheerfulness and good humour. Much statistical matter should have been omitted—'tables which contain the statistics of each county, the produce of the mines, the culture of the vine, and mode of preparing Tokay, and the quantity of corn grown . . .'—but if the reader wished to learn of the rural economy of Hungary, he 'will find in the work before us every detail' he can desire. The reviewer thought that the most popular parts of the volume would be the two chapters on Vienna. Curiously, he made no mention of Bright's drawings, which remain an attractive feature of the book.

The reviewer's general impression would, I think, be endorsed by most readers of today.

BIBLIOGRAPHY

Dictionary of National Biography. 1886 Richard Bright, Vol. 6, p. 334. Oxford
   University Press.
Cameron, H. C. Richard Bright at Guy's, *Guy's Hosp. Rep.* **107**, 263 (1958).
Chance, Burton. Richard Bright, traveller and artist. *Bull. Hist. Med.* 8, 909
   (1940).
Garrison, F. H. Richard Bright's travels in lower Hungary; a physician's
   holiday. *Bull. Johns Hopkins Hosp.* **23**, 173 (1912).
Honti, J. Richard Bright, Edward Brown, and John Paget's travels in Hungary.
   Int. Cong. Hist. Med. **1**, 690 (1972).
Kark, R. M. and Moore, D. T. The life, work, and geological collections of
   Richard Bright, MD (1789–1858); with a note on the collections of other
   members of the family. *Archs Nat. Hist.* **10**, 119 (1981).
Williamson, R. T. Richard Bright; his early travels. *Br. Med. J.* ii, 67 (1927).

10

Clarke Abel in China: 1816–1817

CLARKE ABEL was Surgeon to the second British Embassy which travelled to China in 1816. I have not been able to discover anything of his medical training, but the title page of his book—*Narrative of a Journey in the interior of China*—published in 1819, indicates that he was an MD, a Fellow of the Royal Society and of the Linnean Society, and a member of the Geological Society. He was thirty years of age when he was appointed to the embassy, and his degree of MD was awarded by the University of St. Andrews in 1819, in which year he was made FRS. His testimonials at St. Andrews were signed by Robert Gooch and William King, both of London, stating that he had 'attended a complete course of lectures in the several branches of medicine' but not specifying where. There is a reference to his also being an MRCS, in Crawford's *Roll of the Indian Medical Service*. In an obituary in the *Gentleman's Magazine* (1827, 2, 644) he was praised for his account of the geology of the Cape of Good Hope, and for his service in Calcutta, where he died in 1826.

The first British Embassy to China, in 1793, was led by Earl Macartney, who had already carried out a mission to Russia in 1764. He subsequently became the Governor of the Cape of Good Hope. The mission to the Emperor in Peking sought to open up commercial relations, but, like the second, it was a failure. The Emperor and his court reckoned they possessed all things of value; new things and inventions were not welcomed. Gifts were interpreted as tributes from an inferior people and were rejected. There was the famous coach, in which the coachman was placed inside so that the Emperor could ride outside 'on the nearest seat to heaven'.

The second embassy, arranged when European peace had been restored, and when there was a new emperor in Peking, was also sent with the object of developing trade.

For many years English merchants in Canton had been complaining of the injustices and exactions on the part of the Chinese mandarins. In the sixteenth century the Portuguese and their Jesuits had voyaged to

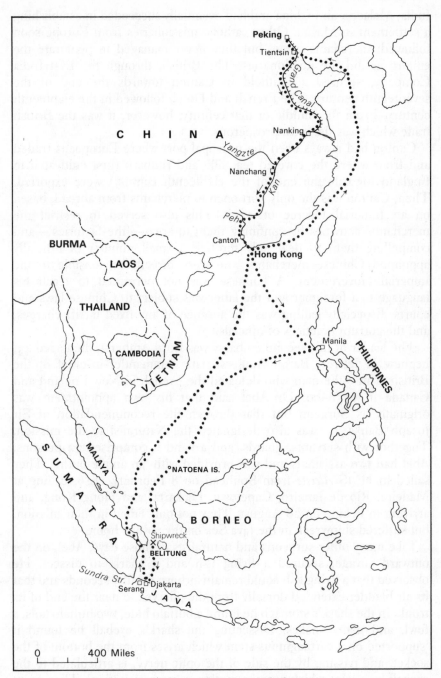

CLARKE ABEL IN CHINA, 1816-17

India, Malacca, and China and had eventually succeeded in establishing a settlement in Macao. Other catholic missionaries from Europe soon followed; merchants came, but they never managed to penetrate the empire as did the missionaries. The British, through the East India Company, secured a foothold in Canton towards the end of the seventeenth century. The French and Dutch followed in the eighteenth century. From the middle of that century, however, it was the British trade which was the most prosperous.

Canton had always been the principal port where Europeans traded and from where the coveted tea, silk, and rhubarb (first cultivated in England towards the end of the eighteenth century) were exported. Then, Canton was the only port open to merchants from abroad, based on an Imperial Decree of 1757. This also served to restrict the merchants' activities by confining them to areas—'the factories'—and compelling them to deal only through a small number of officially appointed Chinese merchants who were directly responsible to the Imperial Government. A Chinese was not permitted to teach his language to a foreigner and the latter was subject to Chinese laws and courts. Especially galling was the absence of any fixed tarriff charges, and the corrupt practices of officials.

The leader of this second embassy was Lord Amherst, then aged 43, nephew of Jeffrey, Baron Amherst, late commander-in-chief of the British army—the man who defeated the French in New England and Canada in 1758–60. Dr Abel said that his own appointment was originally as Surgeon but that through the recommendation of Sir Joseph Banks, he was also designated the Naturalist to the mission. Together with servants, guards, and a band it comprised 72 persons. Abel had two assistants and was provided with 'an ample outfit'. They sailed in HMS *Alceste* from Spithead on 8 February 1816, calling at Madeira, Rio de Janeiro, Capetown, Djakarta, and Hong Kong, and arriving in Peking on 28 August. They not only failed in their mission, but suffered shipwreck in the Java Sea on the voyage home.

Like many other surgeons and naturalists of those days, Abel, on the outward voyage, secured a flying fish and a shark, to dissect. He observed that a flying fish could remain airborn for fifty seconds and that its air bladder extended dorsally from the pharynx to near the end of its trunk. In the shark's stomach he found a buffalo hide, two buffalo tails, a fowl, and many snakes. Dissecting the shark's eyeball he found it 'supported on a cartilaginous stem which arises from the bottom of the socket, and passing by the side of the optic nerve, is articulated to the eyeball by a joint which permits motion in every direction'. They spent two weeks in Java, travelling overland from Anyer Point to Djakarta, while the *Alceste* passed through the Sunda Strait. Abel examined the anatomy of a sucking fish, a bat, and a boa constrictor. He saw the snake swallow a live duck and aboard ship, on the voyage home, he saw a boa seize hold of a goat's leg, strangle it in eight minutes and then proceed to swallow it. This took him two hours—there were great gulping and inspiratory movements, the goats horns almost protruded through his skin and the snake's diameter doubled. Afterwards, it slept for three days.

In the mountains South of Djakarta his geological interests took him up to the crater of one of the many volcanoes in the region and in the adjacent islands. (The *Alceste* passed close to the island of Krakatoa in the Sunda Strait, which was almost completely destroyed by the eruption of 1883). Abel found the mountain people friendly and helpful; he admired their skill in working straw, bamboo, and wood, and the many uses they found for different vegetable oils. Their ornaments and arms were beautifully made and decorated—especially the kriss, the dagger with the wavy blade.

The voyage through the South China Sea to Hong Kong took them twenty days. Although typhoons threatened at times, nothing uneventful happened except for a sting Abel sustained when he picked up what he thought was a piece of floating seaweed 'with an air bubble'. It turned out to be a specimen of *Physalia*, the Portuguese man o'war or bluebottle and for five minutes he had a pain in an armpit followed by a sense of constriction in his chest which lasted fifteen minutes.

In the three days they spent in Hong Kong, he came to realize its future importance for shipping, but he did not consider its scenery in any way picturesque. There were high conical-shaped mountains, deep ravines and rushing torrents, and barren rocks. The miserable inhabitants lived in mud huts and subsisted on fish and the few patches of rice, yam and buck-wheat which they managed to cultivate.

Another two weeks sailing through the East China Sea and the Yellow Sea, brought them to the mouth of the river Pei-ho below Tientsin. Here, two mandarins came aboard to welcome them; they were tall, stately and robust and enjoyed the cherry brandy they were offered. The English were to find that this was 'the most seducing cordial' which could be offered to any Chinese palate. In the ensuing week there was much coming and going of mandarins and officials; junks arrived to take off the presents intended for the Emperor, the band played, and there were entertainments. Abel said the mandarins smelled of a mixture of garlic and asafoetida, and they were constantly spitting. They carried long pipes, and in sheaths around their waists, hung flints and steels used for their smoking, not daggers. The English were always referred to as 'horse-faced men', because of their long faces and large noses.

At last, leaving the *Alceste*, they were transferred to barges and conducted up the river to Tientsin. It was a marshy, unattractive countryside, with dismal huts on the muddy banks and little cultivation; they saw a boy riding downstream, astride a bundle of straw; an occasional dead body floated by. Abel said it was not a particularly inviting 'entrance into China'. After three days on the river they reached Tientsin where they were entertained to 'a feast' during which a play was performed and tumblers cavorted about. The four courses of their meal consisted of soup 'of mare's milk and blood'; sixteen dishes of fruits and dried meats; eight basins of stewed shark's fin, bird's nests, harts' sinews and 'other viands used by the Chinese for their supposed aphrodial virtues'; and twelve bowls of chopped meats floating in gravy. Warm rice wine was drunk from porcelain cups, refilled from small earthenware kettles by servants who bent on one knee.

But it was here that difficulties began. They were not unexpected as they knew of Macartney's experience. The mandarins explained that the English visitors presented to the Emperor would have to perform the ceremonial 'kowtow'. This required them to kneel nine times and touch their foreheads to the ground. Amherst refused and at the Tientsin dinner, when the Chinese brought in some imperial insignia, and performed the kowtow before the English, Amherst simply bowed nine times. During the rest of the journey up river the argument went on, but Amherst promised that he would only bow. At T'ung chow, 13 miles from Peking, they left their boats, more imperial commissioners arrived at their head quarters, and renewed attempts were made to persuade them to perform the full ceremony of kowtowing to the Emperor. But Amherst would have none of it.

Finally, after several days, the English were conducted to a crudely paved road to the Capital. They set out at 4 p.m., the ambassador in a barouche, and the rest of his embassy in sedans, carts, and on horseback; some remained at T'ung chow. The primitive saddles, the spokeless wheels and the jarring of the paved way and the walking pace of the procession, gradually exhausted everyone. They did not arrive in Peking till after midnight. But no sooner had they reached their apartments in a palace, where mandarins, princes, and eunuchs swarmed around them, examining their clothes and equipment, than 'they wanted to bundle the Ambassador into the Emperor's presence in the Imperial Palace'. Suspecting he was being intimidated, and wretchedly worn out, Amherst refused to present himself. There was much noise and confusion and the English finally decided to quit the palace, and using their whips to clear a passage, they went to other English quarters in a village called Hai-teen.

The next morning, Abel felt that the past two days had seemed like a dream. 'The Emperor was incensed at our refusal to see him last night and commanded our immediate departure.' So off they went in procession again down that rough road to T'ung chow and their boats. Several carts overturned and there were casualties; one of the British servants was severely concussed. But they now began to receive messages from the Emperor that some of his ministers had deceived him; he had not understood that Amherst only wished to defer the audience until the next morning. The Emperor sent gifts of precious stones, silk purses, and an agate necklace. Amherst sent portraits of the King and Queen, several engravings, some maps of China, and a painting of Doncaster Races. But there was no question of returning to Peking and in the few days they spent in T'ung chow, Abel roamed around in its suburbs, not being allowed within its walls, observing the people in their shops and stores and saloons. While they smoked their long bamboo pipes, they played at cards or dominoes, and various forms of gambling. Dysentery attacked the British and one died.

Their journey out of China began on 2 September, but not by the way they had entered. Instead, they were conducted to Tientsin, and then by boat down the Grand Canal to Chinkiang and Nanking. Entering the Yangtze river they went southwestwards to Lake Poyang, and then on via the river Kan towards the mountain pass of Meling; climbing this, they went down to Canton on the river Peh. A journey which took them four months. Abel does not make it clear whether they had any choice of route or whether they simply had to do what they were told.

In Tientsin he had opportunity to visit the lapidary shops where he saw many beautiful examples of jade—white, green, blue and yellow—a fondness for which was almost universal in China, though much of the mineral was imported from Burma. Years would be spent on carving a piece after careful study. It was primarily used for producing ornaments and decorative pieces—rings, amulets, chains, cups, vases, and animal figures. Interesting also were the barbers with their range of instruments; they not only shaved the scalp, sparing only the crown, but 'every straggling bit of hair was removed—especially from the ears, nostrils and eyebrows'. The barber would also attend to your corns, pare your nails, and give you a massage. From Tientsin, which they left on 8 September, their boats and barges were mainly towed, not sailed; 'the trackers' who

did the towing were 'miserable-looking men' who were confined at night
to prevent desertion, and who usually sang in chorus as they towed, led
by one man. A popular tune was called 'Pull Away'; its last verse
expressed hope 'for a breakfast in a town'. A few days after starting, and
after a long walk in the sun, Abel fell ill. 'I was attacked by a sudden
affection of the brain which confined me to bed for several weeks.' He
did not describe his symptoms but presumably headache was a feature;
we can deduce from his journal that he did not actually leave his boat to
walk again until they had reached Nanchang—that is, for a period of ten
weeks during which they passed down the canal, the Yangtze, and Lake
Poyang. His observations were thus at first confined to what he saw on
the flat and often inundated countryside. There were villages and towns,
pagodas and temples, rice fields, sluices, flood-gates, swamps, houses on
stilts, old bridges and rock carvings, a variety of masts and sails—and
everywhere, peasants and soldiers. He thought the Yangtze, flowing
from west to east across the land of China, was one of the finest rivers of
the Old World.

At Nanking, the former capital, he was able to see its 200 foot,
nine-storeyed, octagonal-shaped tower of porcelain. The walled city
stood on a hill and no one from the embassy was allowed to enter. The
walls were so famous that there was a Chinese saying that if two
horsemen started at daybreak to gallop around them in opposite
directions, they would not meet till sunset. On the outskirts of another
riverside town there were long rows of 'retiring houses . . . constructed
for exposure rather than concealment'. They consisted of a series of
open sheds where people went to defecate; a rail ran across the
necessary reservoir. The human manure was dried, cut into slabs a foot
square and a few inches thick; it was then odourless. From such
'factories, these slabs, now smelling like violets', were transported to
various parts of the country. It was a thriving industry.

As they approached Lake Poyang the countryside grew more
interesting; there were more hills, and woods of oak and firs. But they
lost a British guard when he fell into a river and drowned. To the west of
the lake they saw snow-covered mountains; the crossing was boisterous.
At one place on the shore there were the ruins of an old national
seminary, all carvings and archways set in a romantic background, in a
green ravine. Once a thriving city it was now deserted but for beggars. In
Nanchang, where Abel was on his feet again, he delighted in its
celebrated porcelain. 'I scarcely recollect seeing any spectacle in China
that gratified me more than a first-rate porcelain warehouse.' He did not
approve, however, of some of the intimate carvings on vases and

cups—'Exposed and handled in a most open manner . . . and giving us the lowest opinion of Chinese sentiments and decency'. On the banks of the Kan there were many interesting trees and shrubs which he examined and it was here that he made sketches of the simple but ingenious wooden machines used for extracting oils from them.

Approaching the mountains and the upper reaches of the Kan, they encountered rocky shoals and cataracts. The boatmen asked for more money and stopped to pray in a temple. 'It was difficult', Abel said, 'but not dangerous'. At Nankang they left their boats and continued their journey overland—across the 1000 foot mountain pass of Meling. On horseback and in sedan chairs, with capable porters and lively horses, they wound their way up in a long procession on a roughly paved road. Travelling in the opposite direction was a large gang of sweating porters who were actually carrying two fire-engines—presents for the Emperor. The engines were slung on poles with the wheels clear of the ground for fear of damage. Abel does not tell us where the engines originated—but presumably he would have if they had been British. At the top of the pass was an arched gateway inscribed with provincial boundaries. They came down to a plain in four hours, through a landscape of rocky shapes and pyramids of compact limestone.

They were met by soldiers in clean simple uniforms of white and red piping. They had bows and arrows and a few match-locks which they supported on crossed sticks when firing. They looked smarter than any other soldiers they had seen, but the British group were startled when a whole regiment was lined up, and on command, saluted them by falling on their knees, clapping their hands and 'uttering a dismal howl'. They were conducted to the city of Kukong where another fleet of boats was organized to take them down the river Peh to Canton. Christmas Day was celebrated, presumably on the river passage, and they arrived in Canton on New Years Day, 1817. They were welcomed by the English merchants and sailors from the *Alceste*, which had come up the river to meet them. They had had to fire on certain Chinese forts to do so. For the past months the *Alceste* had been busy charting the Chinese coast.

At a reception in Canton the Chinese Viceroy, who was distinctly uncooperative, 'grew pale and his eyes sunk under the stern and steady gaze of the English Ambassador'. Once more, the British were not permitted to enter the city proper, whose gates were constantly guarded. They had to satisfy themselves in exploring its suburbs and the local countryside. The skilfully made wares of tortoisehell and ivory, rock crystal and agate, filled their shops. There were exquisitely delicate fans, mirror glass cut as thin as writing paper, spectacle lenses, and lacquered woods. Corundum and adamantine spar were used as cutting tools. Apothecary shops were stocked with an extraordinary variety of medicinal preparations, complete in packets with instructions. Camphor, mercury, and vegetable oils were very popular. Opium was not sold in the shops; it was still contraband but used everywhere in tobacco. (The importation of opium by the British, from India, was alarming the Chinese authorities and ultimately led to the 'Opium War' in 1841–42.) Abel observed the addict's 'peculiar, sotish, sleepy physiognomy'. The medical men he met had little idea of human anatomy; they new of the heart, lungs, liver, spleen, and kidneys but little about their actual location. He showed them an anatomical illustration in a volume of the *Encyclopaedia Brittanica* he found in the library of the English factory. One Chinese doctor said it would be the best imaginable gift to distribute in the land. [But it would have had to compete with the various versions of the Bible then circulating.] Vaccination was being introduced by one of the English doctors. Itinerant Chinese practitioners used the moxa method to produce counterirritation; the affected part was often pierced with a gold pin and dried Artemesia leaves were the most popular source of the powder which would be ignited on the skin. Abel was told that in Northern China ignition was often produced by using 'a convex mirror of ice'. Many Chinese bore scars from these treatments.

In the gardens, azaleas, camellias, and roses flourished and Abel learned how dwarf plants were grown—in pots too small for their roots, with branches tied in curves, and the bark wounded to give the appearance of age. Like all Englishmen Abel was highly interested in the Chinese 'Tcha' or 'Tea' which had appeared in England in the seventeenth century, and had become a monopoly of the East India Company. Abel wondered whether it could be cultivated in Capetown or Rio. Trading with China presented so many difficulties that the British had to develop an independent supply but this they were not able to do—in Assam—until the 1830's. Abel's friend, Sir Joseph Banks, had originally suggested the location. Abel wondered also whether there was any difference between black and green tea. He visited plantations, observed methods of drying and fermentation, and came to the conclusion, correctly, that in making the green variety, the leaf is subjected to heat which prevents fermentation. There was no species difference.

He also watched local printers at work with wooden blocks; at that time only the *Peking Gazette* used movable type. But all Chinese towns looked the same, he wrote, if you had seen one town or pagoda you had seen them all. The temples and their grotesque idols, gilded monsters, lighted tapers, paper prayers, tolling bells, dormitories and labyrinths, and costumed bronzes—did not excite any feeling of appreciation for their philosophy and religions. The peasants were friendly and helpful, the merchants greedy, and he regretted that he had but little intercourse with the educated classes.

They all sailed away in the *Alceste* on 20 January, made a short call at Macao to see the English factory, and then turned southwards to Manila, in the Philippines, where they were well received by the Spanish governor. Arriving on 2 February, in the middle of a festival in honour of the Blessed Virgin, Abel watched some of the processions and was prompted to comment that, after just witnessing several Chinese religious occasions—'I could not but regret that the ministers of the pure religion of Christ, and those of the vilest idolatry which disgraces human nature, should endeavour by like methods to influence the minds of the people'. The Spanish colony looked to be a rich place; the majority of the people were half-castes, many of them handsome; they wore fine clothes and there were plenty of good carriages. The Governor's palace was protected by fortification and a drawbridge. Everyone smoked large cigars, even the women in the streets. They were usually six to eleven inches in length, and one and a half inches in diameter, so that 'the mouth seems scarcely large enough to grasp them'. The Chinese were disliked and watched. One day in the square, Abel saw three men executed; they were garrotted by means of an iron collar and a large screw which was suddenly turned. At the end of a gay evening of dining, dancing, and merrymaking, our stern hero was tempted to admit that perhaps after all there was something to be said for miscegenation—'Olla podrida was not the least attractive ornament'.

One evening they were taken to see some celebrated hot springs in the jungle. They were rowed in a felucca by 16 men to a lake where they rested and had a supper of fowls and wine in a convent. The friar was plump and jovial. They reached the springs at 6 a.m., where there was another convent. Here, their host was a comic little man with a big head covered with a shock of black hair, a wide mouth, and thick lips, who came running out barefeet with his shirt hanging out beneath an old-fashioned black jacket. He grinned amiably, circling each visitor in turn, inspecting them minutely. The embassy chaplain, a double-shotgun in his hands, was introduced as a fellow cleric. This caused their host great amazement and he promptly darted indoors and soon returned with a fresh shirt, stockings, and buckled shoes. A woman was called, tall, dark, and thin, who poured them delicious chocolate and large goblets of the coldest water. She reminded Abel of the Indian wife of Lieutenant Lismahago in Tobias Smollett's *Humphry Clinker*. The hot springs were in the clearance in the jungle, surrounded by exotic shrubs and plants. There were bamboo floors to walk over them and some had dome-shaped, thatched roofs. The waters bubbled out at 174 °F and the steam was at 108 °F. Rivulets winded their way in and out among the rocks and foliage, and the trees seemed enwrapped by swirling coloured vapours. Abel was reluctant to leave such a novel scene. Back at the convent they dined well, served by young females who remained standing and smiling in the cool room. Abel was highly intrigued by their presence.

They left Manila the following day and sailed southwards, passing the Natoena Islands on 16 February, and running for 160 miles on the 17th. Abel was up early on the 18th to see their passage through the straits between the islands of Bangka and Belitung in the Java Sea. Suddenly, as he stood on deck, he felt a giant shudder pass through the ship, and a loud rumbling noise. They had struck a coral reef, heeled over slightly to starboard, and settled.

It soon became evident that they would have to lower their boats and abandon ship. The Ambassador and one party rowed three miles to an uninhabited island. Others followed, but the ship's captain and a few officers and crew remained aboard for the day and following night. After exploring around in the creeks of the island, and finding no source of fresh water, they spent most of the time salvaging what they could from the sinking vessel. They built a camp, slung a hammock in the trees for Amherst, lit fires and set up guards for the night. It was a notorious area for pirates. Next morning Abel went back to the *Alceste* to see if he could save his trunk of minerals, plants, and seeds. It was placed on a raft but subsequently set on fire by Malays. Returning to the camp he joined the barge in which the Ambassador and thirty-three others proposed to try to sail and row to Djakarta. They were accompanied by a cutter carrying seventeen others. The remainder of the company—190 in all—armed with 40 muskets, 40 boarding pikes, and 20 cutlasses, stayed on the island, making preparations to defend themselves. They were told that help would be sent as soon as possible.

The barge and cutter reached Djakarta four days later—the survivors exhausted, blistered, and dehydrated and with one man delirious from drinking sea water. Two British vessels were in the harbour and they set off to rescue the others on the following morning. The first ship arrived in the nick of time; Malayan pirates had looted and burned the *Alceste*, attacking the British, who were forced to retreat and fortify a hill on the island. Abel said there were 'four to five hundred Malayan prows' assembled for a final assault when HMS *Termate* arrived on the scene. All the survivors were brought back to Djakarta.

Abel spent seven weeks there and appears not to have suffered serious harm although he found the city a most unhealthy and unlovely place—which it still is. Built on swampy soil close to the sea, Abel was 'astonished at the infinite pains that have been taken to unite in one spot all the causes of disease'. There were numerous dirty intersecting canals, discarded refuse, floating carcasses, and poorly ventilated houses whose doors and windows the Dutch kept closed throughout the day. 'It was the grave of many thousand Europeans.' He was equally astonished by the way European men persisted in wearing their national dress, whereas the ladies sensibly adopted the native types of loose cotton robes (presumably sarongs). But both sexes ate and drank too much, and spent much of the day asleep. At night they consumed gargantuan meals. An English cantonment a few miles outside the town was healthier and better regulated.

As a naturalist, he devoted many pages of his journal to an account of the fruits, shrubs and trees he studied. From the Dutch Governor's summer residence in the hills, he enjoyed walking in the forests, and watching the spectacular storms, and collecting specimens. He sampled most of the exotic fruits, finding the taste of the mangosteen 'between pineapple and peach' and the odour of the esteemed durian, like 'sulphuretted hydrogen'. Particularly gorgeous were the galaxies of hibiscus and poinsettias.

They began their voyage home on 12 April, in HMS *Caesar*, taking with them for the London Zoological Garden, a boa constrictor and a young orang outang. They coped with a fire, south of Mauritius, and arrived at the Cape of Good Hope on 27 May. In two weeks there, Abel the geologist, spent most of his time studying the rock formation, devoting thirty pages of his journal to its description, and later lecturing on the subject to his colleagues in London. For the pundit, his findings were 'illustrative and confirmative of the theories of Hutton and Werner'. Two days at St Helena in late June afforded an opportunity of a fifteen-minute audience with Napoleon Bonaparte whom he observed to be well and active—'in excellent plight'. There was something very impressive about his gaze, posture, and movements, but afterwards the British officers could not agree on the colour of his eyes. Napoleon died, it will be remembered, in 1821, of cancer of the stomach. A turtle which Abel caught on the rat-infested Ascension Island, proved to be a source of anxiety to the orang-outang. The physical characteristics of the latter were carefully described by him. Two feet seven inches in height, he chased about the rigging with the sailors, jumped into their arms, picked their pockets for food and went to sleep at the masthead, wrapped in a sail. He preferred tea and coffee to wine or beer, and by the time they arrived at Spithead on 16 July, he had learned to eat with a spoon.

When Abel's journal was published a year later, the botanist Robert Brown, librarian to Sir Joseph Banks, and later to become the first keeper of the botanical department of the British Museum, dedicated a genus, *Abelia*, in his honour, founded on one of the plants from China. Subsequently Abel was appointed physician to Lord Amherst when he was made governor-general of India, and he died there in 1826.

11

Thomas Hodgkin in Morocco
1863–1864

To Victorian eyes the scene depicted by the artist may not have looked unfamiliar. It could have been another vignette of Empire, perhaps from the pages of the *Illustrated London News*—a military parley, a diplomatic visit, or a trade mission. There was a large, sunlit but treeless courtyard, within an arcaded Moorish-looking fort, and lined by columns of dark-skinned soldiers, mounted or on foot. They wore turbans and baggy trousers, and carried long scimitars. Flags few. In the centre foreground, on a richly-saddled big white horse, sat a dark-faced man in ornamental headdress and flowing robes, his head turned towards a tall, uniformed figure standing stiffly beside the horse. He appears to be reading from an address he holds in his hands. To the right is grouped an escort of alert-looking, armed natives. On the left is another group of men, but they are white and bare-headed, and wear western dress, frock-coats or uniforms. One of them is small and bearded. Behind them, again, is a pair of horses with a sedan chair slung between them and an attendant at the reins. Further to the left, in the background, is a four-wheeled, horse-drawn carriage, canopied and decorated with fringed trappings.

It was clearly an occasion of some significance. The artist who recorded it was Dr Thomas Hodgkin, possibly the small bearded figure. The soldierly-looking figure at the horse's side represents his friend Sir Moses Montefiore Bart, and the horseman himself was the Emperor of Morocco, Sultan Mohammed XVII. The year was 1864, and it was seven-o-clock in the morning of the first day of February. The illustration itself comes from Hodgkin's posthumously published book entitled *Narrative of a journey to Morocco in 1863 and 1864* (Plate 29).

In 1864 Hodgkin was sixty-five and Montefiore seventy-nine; the one a Quaker physician, the other a Jewish Financier. The doctor was small and slim, the magnate tall (six feet three inches) and heavy. Hodgkin was an ascetic type, scholarly and unworldly, rigid in his views. Montefiore, by all accounts, was gregarious and friendly, very much a man of the world. He lived well, in a fine mansion, and is said to have enjoyed a bottle of port a day until two years before his death at the age of one hundred and one years, in 1885. A curiously assorted pair, many have said. However, they were both devout and philanthropic and for forty years this was the probable basis for their friendship, Hodgkin also being the personal physician.

Hodgkin was born in London in 1798. He did not go to school but was tutored by his father, entering Guy's Hospital as a pupil in 1819, and graduating MD in Edinburgh in 1823. He spent some time on the Continent, travelling in France, Germany and Italy and on his return, advocating the use of Laennec's stethoscope. Like Richard Bright he was an accomplished linguist and he was also well-versed in the classics. In 1825 he was appointed lecturer in morbid anatomy and curator of the museum in the newly-opened Guy's medical school. He held this appointment for twelve years, resigning in 1837, when he failed to secure an appointment as physician to Guy's Hospital. He had also been in practice as a physician but he disliked payment by fee and his practice was reputed to have been small, declining as he became involved in other activities. In 1836 he had refused to accept an invitation to become a Fellow of the Royal College of Physicians on the repeal of its bye-law that Fellows must be graduates of Oxford or Cambridge, and, accordingly, members of the Established Church. He wore Quaker dress, and spoke and wrote in the Quaker fashion. One of his published lectures, that on his original account of aortic incompetence in 1829, began with the words 'Thou wilt probably recollect . . .' and he signed his portrait on the frontispiece of his book on Morocco, 'Thine sincerely' (Plate 28).

He appears to have been an awkward man of the crusading type, and despite his obvious sincerity and worthiness, not one who would be warmly welcomed by a majority of a hospital staff of that day. His fame came, it will be remembered, after his death, when the term coined by Dr Samuel Wilks—'Hodgkin's disease'—came to be adopted. It originally appeared in 1865, in the *Guy's Hospital Reports*, a few months before Hodgkin left for the Holy Land, with Montefiore, so he may well have seen it before he died there, in Jaffa, in April 1866.

Throughout his life he was a zealous campaigner in many fields. In medicine he advocated reforms in the promotion of health, the training of doctors, and he stressed the importance of records, autopsies, and the examination of the relation between lesions, symptoms, and signs. As well as lecturing on the stethoscope in his early years as a doctor, he later pleaded for the introduction of the metrical system. He was a member of the senate of the newly-founded University of London, a secretary of the Royal Geographical Society and a vigorous opponent of religious or racial discrimination and injustice. The slave, the negro, the aboriginal, the native in a colony or the American indian on a reservation, and the Jews in Europe, the Middle East, and elsewhere—all, from time to time, were objects of his philanthropic endeavours. And it was in aid of Moroccan Jews that he accompanied Montefiore to Marrakesh in 1863. To Montefiore it was one of many similar journeys—to Moscow, Bucharest, Constantinople, and many times to the Holy Land—which he had undertaken. Hodgkin had often travelled with him in Europe and twice went with him to the Holy Land. Montefiore seems to have been exceptionally robust, energetic and masterful in bringing practical assurances and aid to oppressed Jewish communities. One can readily imagine how he would have reacted to the horrors of this century.

THE NARRATIVE

'*Narrative of a journey to Morocco*' might lead a modern reader to expect a description of the country of Morocco and its people, and this is sometimes implied in modern references to his book. But by 'Morocco' was meant 'Marrakesh', then its capital city. European travellers of the day often wrote of the 'City of Morocco' or 'Marocco'. Nowhere, in Hodgkin's book, is there mention of 'Marrakesh'. He visited Tangier, but his travels within the country were restricted to a relatively small area in the west, from the port of entry Essaouira (then called Mogador) to Marrakesh, and a return journey to the port of exit, El Jadida (then called Mazagan). The distance travelled was not more than two-hundred and thirty miles, but at that time, and for men of their age, it must have been quite arduous. They were away from England for four and a half months, from November 1863 to April 1864. We should also note that it was described as a journey 'to' Morocco, and it began in Dover, where the party of travellers assembled.

The title page also states that the 'late' author was MD and FRGS and that the volume contained certain 'geological annotations', a hint perhaps, not only of Hodgkin's interest, but also that a Victorian armchair-traveller might not find in its pages much to rouse his curiosity or to entertain him. The volume was dedicated to Montefiore and in the editor's preface it is explained that Hodgkin had delivered the manuscript a few days before he left England on his last journey to the Holy Land early in 1866. 'It was in a very crude condition' but the author had intended 'to carefully revise the whole'. Whether this would have entailed anything more than a polishing of prose we cannot say, but

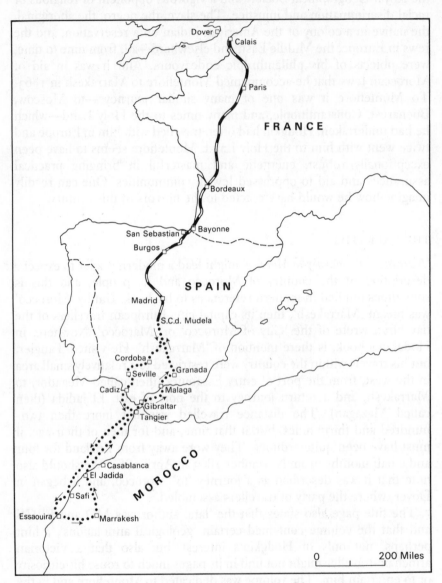

THOMAS HODGKIN IN MOROCCO, 1863–4

judging from its content and style, it is doubtful whether Hodgkin would have recognized that it could have been agreeably enlivened. It is a rather dry travelogue, and even for a Victorian quaker, singularly pedestrian. Montefiore, one feels, could well have provided a leaven of humour and anecdote.

But it was 'a memorial volume', with a portrait of the author, subscribed by his friends and admirers, and with letters of tribute, obituarial notices and an account of his illness and death in Jaffa. From the outset the tone is serious. But then, so also was the reason for the mission.

THE MISSION

The opening lines of the book begin interestingly enough.

On the 31st of 10th month, seventh day, 1863, a packet of letters was received by Sir Moses Montefiore at his country residence, Eastcliffe Lodge, Ramsgate; and as it happened to be his Sabbath, they were all opened for him . . . One of them . . . came from some of the leading members of the Israelitish community of Gibraltar, who were thrown into painful sympathy for their brethren at Tangier, whom recent occurrences had placed in alarm and danger.

It transpired that a Spaniard in government employ in Safi, Morocco, had died suddenly in circumstances which raised a suspicion of foul play. A member of his household, a Jewish boy of fourteen, was arrested and interrogated. He had protested his innocence, but when 'scourged' and 'tortured', as was the Moorish custom, he said that the man had been poisoned and he named ten or eleven Jews who had been involved. They were all arrested and one of them subjected to torture; he did not admit guilt. The boy, meanwhile, when torture had ceased, renewed his protestations of innocence. However, both were sentenced to death, and the boy was publicly executed in Safi. To publicise the alleged Jewish crime, the man was taken to Tangier for execution. The remainder were detained in Safi, 'menaced with a fate like that of their two brethren . . . and there was great dismay among the Jewish population'.

On receipt of the letter, things started to hum in Ramsgate and London. Early the next morning, a Sunday, Montefiore, 'his active benevolence aroused to a high pitch', was off to London, hunting up the Secretary, Earl Russell, and the Under-Secretary, at the Foreign Office. 'In a wonderfully short time the wires of the Continental telegraph were at work', carrying instructions to the British ambassador in Tangier, to do his best to stay any executions. Montefiore arranged with the Jewish

Board of Deputies in London that he should go to Morocco and by 16 November he had assembled a party to accompany him, at the Lord Warden hotel in Dover. There were seven: Montefiore and Hodgkin; a Mr Samuel, solicitor and secretary to the Board of Deputies; a Mr Guedalla, whose father was a merchant in Morocco; a Mr Ferrache, a native of Morocco who had previously assisted Montefiore in his travels; a Mr Oliffe, 'an old and faithful attendant' of the leader; and, lastly, a lady from Hanover, Germany, Albertine Muller, who was 'very familiar with all that can be required, either in sickness or in health, from a female attendant in travel'. One cannot but admire Sir Moses, the 'venerable leader' approaching his eightieth year, and his bold band of friends. They must have been very attached to him.

THE OUTWARD JOURNEY

They crossed to Calais the next morning and stayed the night at Sir Moses's favourite hotel in Paris, Meurice's. They reached Bordeaux by train on the second night and rested there for two days. Montefiore found time to see friends and acquaintances, including the superintendent of the Bordeaux plant belonging to the Imperial Continental Gas Company, of which Montefiore was a founder. The train took them on to Bayonne, across the pine-scented plain of the *Landes* where Hodgkin noted with pleasure the work of reclamation in progress, both in tilling and planting. Cork and turpentine were becoming important exports. There were few examples to be seen of the herdsmen who used stilts in the marshes, and who, when resting on their perches, 'would fill up their leisure hours in knitting stockings'.

Sir Moses was travelling incognito, but a Mr Leon of Bayonne, accosted Hodgkin in the street, and made enquiries of his party. Hodgkin's replies were evasive and he was surprised to find Mr Leon with his party at their hotel, later in the day. He proved to be most helpful. On a visit to 'the little town of Biarritz', Hodgkin was pleased to note that it resembled 'an English watering-place' and with shops which carried English notices. Noticing the door-plate of an English physician, he was emboldened to ring the bell, and discovered the doctor to be 'a very agreable and intelligent gentleman'.

The next stage of their journey, via St. Jean de Luz, and Irun, where they were subjected to 'a long detention' by frontier officials, to San Sebastian, was completed by rail and diligence. There, Hodgkin observed the evening promenaders in their Sunday dress and watched some Basque dancers and musicians. 'Of the dance', he said, 'I could form no opinion'. On the following day the train took them to Burgos; and on the next, to Madrid. On the way, in Avila, Hodgkin was left behind while he had gone sight-seeing. It appeared to him to be a city of granite, with 'a dark and gloomy cathedral'. In Madrid, where they stayed for eight days in the Hotel de los Principes, in 'the most desirable situation in Madrid', Montefiore was busily engaged with the British ambassador, the Prime Minister and others. Despite the assurances he received about the Moroccan Jews, 'he was unwilling to quit Madrid until he had had a personal interview with the Queen herself'. In this he was eventually, and characteristically, successful.

Hodgkin, in the meantime, could not find much to interest him in the city. 'It is not a city which possesses many of the objects which suit my taste.' The museum was closed when he chose to visit, so also was that part of the picture gallery which contained 'the little which is worthy of attention'. The veterinary college had been moved to a new site, and the hospital was closed, 'the hour being late'; an attendant allowed him 'to see some of the wards'. The view of the city and the distant mountains, from the observatory hill, was not 'particularly striking'.

There must be few English travel writers, who had so little to say after a week's stay in Madrid. His two doleful pages should not have passed beyond the editor's desk.

The railroad terminated at the little town of Santa Cruz de Mudela, where they stayed a night. The white-washed houses and streets reminded Hodgkin of Ireland, but instead of windows there were iron grills, and shutters. The women sat at their open doors, sewing or knitting; the men wore rough clothes, and instead of stockings and shoes, 'coarse linen, bound rudely about their legs'. An ass turned a water-wheel. They were in a diligence at five on the next morning. They crossed the Sierra Morena, 'at the summit of which the aneroid barometer stood at 27 inches'. Then, as they descended, the fields were more cultivated and there were many olive groves. They arrived at Andujar at tea-time, and, while Montefiore rested there for the night, Hodgkin and Guedalla went on to Cordoba, arriving about midnight.

It was a large city, on the Guadalquivir, retaining much of its Moorish character. Hodgkin saw the Caliph's palace, then a prison, the market place, the Moorish bridges across the river, and a herd of pigs on its bank, fine and clean, 'not so disgustingly unwieldy and flabby' as the stye-reared English variety. A skin of leather hanging up reminded him that in his youth he used to hear shoe-makers refer to 'Cordevan' leather. He admired the style of the houses and buildings, with their inner, cloistered courtyards, and the flowers and iron grill doors. In the cathedral, with its original mosque construction, 'the eight hundred and sixty columns of marble and granite, forming avenues and supporting arches, produced an effect something like that of a pine forest'. An elephant's tusk, unearthed from the cathedral floor, caused him to wonder whether it was from a native animal or whether it was brought in by the Carthaginians.

He saw the church tomb of 'a celebrated writer, Morales'. This was probably that of Luis De Morales, 'El Divino', the sixteenth century artist. No mention was made of Averroes or Maimonides, the physician-philosophers of twelfth century Cordoba.

A few days later the train took them on to Seville and Cadiz, where they arrived on the 8th of December. They sailed to Tangier on a French frigate on the evening of the 10th, arriving there at five-o-clock next morning. 'Sir Moses's arrival had been anticipated and well prepared for, a large concourse of people being ready to receive him.' In the absence of a pier 'there was a multitude in the water . . . waiting to bear us to the shore'. The sight of the big Montefiore being carried over the water on a couch 'contrived of a mattress and cordage', appeared to Hodgkin, in a rare moment of amusement, 'like a travestied representation of Neptune among the Tritons'.

TANGIER

When they had all been carried ashore by the wading natives, they found themselves surrounded 'by a vast number of Israelite population from the town, of all classes and both sexes'. For the first time, Hodgkin heard 'the peculiar sound uttered by the Jewish females in Morocco when they wish to give expression to their joyful greetings with distinguished honour'. Sir Moses was dissuaded from putting up at 'the best hotel', although run by a Scottish lady. Arrangements had already been made for the party to be accommodated in a fine comfortable house, with courtyard and balconies, vacated by the Jewish owner for the occasion. For the next ten days it was their headquarters.

Sir Moses received deputations from the Jews of Tetuan, Alcazar (El Ksar), El Kebir, Arzila (Asilah), Laraish (Larache) and Mequinez (Meknes), and addresses from Mogador (Essaouira), Azamor (Azemmour), and Fez. He attended the synagogue and visited the British and Spanish embassies and talked with the Moorish Minister for Foreign Affairs. Two of the Jews in Tangier jail were released and came to thank him. What is more, fifty Moors from 'a distant part of the country' came to Sir Moses to ask his help in obtaining the release from jail of one of their tribe who had been accused of murdering two Jews, and held without trial for two-and-a-half years. 'In a few hours the prisoner's chains were removed' and he also came to thank Sir Moses. In return the Moors promised that 'all Jews travelling by day should be perfectly safe'.

The Tangier Jews were visited in their homes and entertained at the headquarters. Jewish girls were far more attractive than the Moorish, 'many of them were really beautiful'. They touched up their eyelashes and eyelids with powdered antimony but Hodgkin thought this practice was 'not in the least degree ornamental'. However, although he confessed that he was 'a poor observer and worse describer of female attire', he admired the richly embroidered silk garments they wore, unspoilt 'by the interference of the European fashion of thin iron hoops, known by the inappropriate name of crinoline'. Their head-dresses had 'a brilliant gaiety', and their nails and finger tips were stained nearly black, much darker than the colour from henna, as used in Egypt and Palestine. The most popular jewel was the emerald. Sir Moses made a bequest to start a school for poorer Jewish girls, who, he was told, might suffer educationally, as did Moorish girls.

Hodgkin gave a lecture and conducted some chemical experiments for the young people. With a home-made machine, and using a wine bottle to make a Leyden jar, as he had learned in his youth, he endeavoured to generate an electrical spark. He failed in this and concluded that the bottle had not be blown, but made in a mould, and was not smooth enough for his purpose.

Tangier itself proved interesting. It lay in a valley between two hills which were terraced with white houses. Between them was the town centre, with its main street and market place. In the market, poultry were kept in small cylindrical cages made of reeds; the loaves of bread were large and flat, 'resembling Bath cakes'; there were many varieties of grain, seed, and nuts for sale; dates and other dried fruits were abundant. The local soap resembled 'a tar ointment', and the candles were conical in shape, two-inches at the base, and nearly a foot long. Although the majority of the natives wore 'white woollen Burnous', many were adopting European dress. Wealthier Jews wore 'a kind of tunic, generally blue, and bearing some resemblance to a dressing gown'.

On the western hill was the Governor's residence and official buildings, barracks, prison, and mosques. Through a fine Moorish gateway in the old city wall, there was a view of gardens, fields and woods. About the residences there, were many delightful hanging gardens with views across the water to Spain. Outside the town there were open spaces, pens, and enclosures for horses, cattle, and pigs. Shoeing a horse looked to be a cruel procedure; the hoof was chopped away with a kind of adze, and not paired with a knife. The camels were thin, miserable creatures, unlike those he had seen in Egypt. They were 'sadly wrung and sore' after carrying badly arranged loads from the interior.

GIBRALTAR

They sailed to Gibraltar on 22 December and stayed there for two weeks. As at Tangier, there was great excitement among the Jewish community, and 'good quarters . . . with a capital view of the bay and town', were ready for them. A military band played for them that evening, and later they were all received at Government House. Montefiore was 'zealous and indefatigable' among the Jewish community. Hodgkin, who had previously visited Gibraltar, inspected the galleries which had been cut in the rock by the military. He was taken to see the excavations which had been going on in certain caves. Archaeologists and palaeontologists had been busy; ancient animal and human bones had been discovered. Some had been sent to the Royal College of Surgeons in London. He saw some examples of 'early human art' in one of the caverns.

A naval frigate, HMS *Magicienne*, under the command of a Captain Armytage, 'had been ordered by telegram from England, to proceed from Malta' and convey the party to Safi. Hodgkin made no mention of how he spent Christmas. They steamed off on 6 January, after collecting tents, beds, and cooking pots, 'and all those articles necessary for the overland journey' to Marrakesh. Hodgkin slung his hammock 'between two guns'. They arrived off Safi three days later. The voyage was pleasant and uneventful and 'the nautical operations of the master and sailors, the practice of the midshipmen with their sextants, the guns and other furniture of the ships, afforded abundant source of interest and amusement'.

The weather proved too rough for them to land at Safi, but by signal they learned that the Jewish prisoners had already been released and that a Sultan's escort awaited to conduct them to Marrakesh, 'about one hundred miles distant'. They steamed on through the night, in rough seas, to the port of Essaouria. A reef made navigation into the harbour difficult. Sir Moses was 'lowered in an arm-chair into one of the boats' and taken ashore. Hodgkin was taken in a native boat piloted by an old man who did not stop shouting at the rowers. They also all kept shouting, and rowed by jumping up and down on their seats in a strange fashion.

ESSAOUIRA TO MARRAKESH

In Essaouira, like Safi a former Portuguese port, there were ancient fortifications and cannon, and the city itself was divided into three quarters—Christian, Moorish, and Jewish—each with its own gate which was closed at night. The place was dirty, especially the Jewish quarter. The caravan assembled in an open space, amidst a crowd of spectators. Soldiers, horses, and mules were provided by the government, and there were camels and porters. Sir Moses and Hodgkin found the Moorish saddles very awkward, so they began the journey on foot. A covered sedan-chair, slung between two mules, was provided for Sir Moses; its motion was not pleasant. Many pedestrians and riders accompanied them on the first stage of their journey, including the town governor, the chief Jews, and the French Consul with his wife and family.

The party no longer contained Guedalla and Oliffe; they had left for Nice, to attend the funeral of Montefiore's sister, who died there while they were in Gibraltar. They had been joined by Captain Armytage and Dr Forbes of HMS *Magicienne*, and also by a Mr Fairly, a civil engineer *en route* to Marrakesh. There was also a Mr Reade, Consul at Tangier.

They headed inland, passing a deserted palace, an aqueduct, tombs, and ruins. Hodgkin was soon commenting on the geological features of the countryside, which appeared to remain his chief interest in Morocco. The journey to Marrakesh took nine days. Hodgkin's mule was 'a wretched beast', and the saddle was very uncomfortable. He walked when he could, but the ground was often stony and crossed by wadis. They had to ford several streams and rivers, some of which had steep banks and pebbly beds. A baggage mule fell in one stream and was only rescued with difficulty. Mr Samuel also fell from his mule and 'his nerves were shaken'.

They rose early each day, stopped for an hour or so for lunch, and were usually pitching their camp by nightfall. Sometimes the going was fair, over flat and sandy tracks. Hodgkin's illustration of an encampment shows that their caravan must have been quite a lengthy one. Fourteen tents may be seen, over one of which flies the Union Jack; there are many camels, mules, and horses; dozens of natives; and on the left of the picture, two sedan-chairs, one, the larger, presumably Sir Moses's, as Hodgkin said it was a sort of 'wooden house or sedan'. On one occasion it nearly overturned. It was hot by day, often very cold at night, with heavy dews. There were no serious mishaps or illnesses. They often camped near a village stream or well, many of the latter being obviously ancient and deep. The villagers pulled up the vessels 'with long cords which had worn the sides, as we may see in the marble mouths of wells in Italy'. In one well the grooves were four inches deep, 'which indicates great antiquity, for the stone—a buff and pink limestone, resembling Sicilian jasper—is very hard'. The water was usually cold and pure, but at one well it had 'a very decided sulphurous odour, like that of St. Bernard's well, near Leith'. They also came across covered, underground cisterns, usually on the rock slopes of a hill.

Near Marrakesh, after crossing the river Tensift, there were several subterranean aqueducts. Lines of earth mounds marked the sites of vertical pits which had been excavated. 'The bottom of these pits communicated with each other by lateral shafts . . .' as he had seen in London when water pipes were being laid down. But here the channels were too big and unlined so that there was an 'incalculable amount of waste of water'. Outside Marrakesh there was a well-built aqueduct, a few feet above ground level.

The general management of the caravan, the loading and unloading, the erection of tents and the preparation of food, all improved as they progressed, and Captain Armytage was particularly helpful. At times, 'with the ground well trodden and strewn with litters' the scene reminded Hodgkin of the breaking up of a fair site.

The indigenous Berbers were friendly and curious as they met them in the villages and markets, or in their 'large brown tents' in the countryside. There were no dangerous incidents, but once, a native drew a knife and demanded money from a few of their advance party. When others came up 'a strong soldier gave him twenty lashes on the bare back, with a leather rope. The man afterwards kissed the knees of the soldier and was lead away by his people.'

At certain stages they would be met by a chief or his emissaries, who would present them with gifts, 'a mona'. Once, they were given 'three or four sheep, many fowls, one thousand eggs, melons, a stupendous gourd, honey, ten pounds of loaf sugar, wax or composite candles, vegetables etc. . . .'. On another occasion, the mona being scanty, Consul Reade complained to the village chief 'who was made a prisoner the next morning; but he in his turn complained of one of his men, and gave him a beating'. Midway to Marrakesh, a courier arrived from the city; he had taken seventy hours on foot. He told them that a gunpowder magazine had blown up there and that 'six or eight hundred lives had been lost'.

One morning after breakfast they were given a display of horsemanship by a company of soldiers from a provincial governor. They watched them 'dashing abreast, after galloping at a rapid pace for about two hundred yards, fired simultaneously at the ground, and then raising their long guns in the air, quickly stopped'. Many a modern tourist has since captured this spectacle with his camera. One chief had 'a French double-barrelled rifle' with which a companion executed a drill which one of the party 'recognised as being of the French school'.

Moroccan horses, Hodgkin observed, were the best in North Africa, although he acknowledged that those of Arabia 'had the most poetical and world-wide celebrity'. Moroccan 'barbs' were 'the ancestors of the best horses of which England can boast'; They had fine crests and hind-quarters, with large low hocks. They were very strong, 'capable of carrying twelve stones . . . they could gallop a mile in two minutes'.

They saw many 'castellated buildings enclosed by walls' [Kasbahs], ruined dwellings among which tents were pitched or huts erected, and often a surround of high prickly bushes. There were sheep, cattle, and goats; corn and seed; and dark honeycombs in the village markets. There were signs of ancient irrigation and building, but Hodgkin never found any fragments of pottery. Where there was alluvial soil, rude ploughs were used, drawn by a variety of animals—horse, ass, cow, oxen, or camel—sometimes in combination. At one camp where there was a good stream, a pool contained fish. 'There was a pretty copse, as well as two or three palm trees.' Captain Armytage shot some snipe which they had for supper; the partridges 'were too wild to be had'. Elsewhere, they saw duck, small game fowl, turkeys, pigeons, plover, ravens, and 'poules de Carthage', a small species of bustard. Storks' nests were identified about mosques and kasbahs, but although there were packages of ostrich feathers at Essaouira, they saw no birds or eggs. One bird which was as esteemed as the stork, was called 'the cow-bird'. Larger than a crow, it was milky-white, with small eyes and a light, yellow-coloured beak; it was quiet and gregarious. Although clearly not water-fowls, they liked to collect near pools and streams.

At times, white broom scented the air, and there were liliaceous plants, euphoria, and crocuses in abundance. On the banks of some streams grew oleanders, and they saw a plantation of prickly pears. Cultivation was scanty, in patches, and trees were small; there were many scattered clumps of thorny bush. In one place, what looked from a distance to be white blossom, turned out to be a species of small white snail on the leafless boughs of shrubs and trees. Olive groves were not seen in this part of their journey, but there was a tree called 'argand', of a beautiful green colour and producing a valuable oil. (These trees, still to be seen along the Atlantic coast, are said to be peculiar to Morocco and parts of South America; their oil is used for cooking.)

The physical geography of this part of western Morocco—the ancient kingdom of Marrakesh, was of great interest to geologically-minded Hodgkin. There is not only much description of the features of the ground over which they passed, its surface, outcrops, hills, cliffs, ravines, and terraces, but, in a twenty-two page addendum there is a detailed account of 'some superficial geological appearances'. To anyone without this particular interest, it is rather boring, but it nevertheless displays the sharpness of his eye and keenness of his curiosity. And, as we shall see, some of his findings, 'hitherto, I believe, altogether unnoticed', were of great significance.

On the coast, with its dunes and puce-coloured sandstone cliffs, he commented on the erosion and the effects of inward-sweeping sands. He soon began to see evidence of extensive and remarkable formations of limestone, and continued to do so on the journey to and from Marrakesh. He said it resembled the limestone which he had seen 'between Rome and Tivoli, and called travertin', a porous light yellow rock, hardening on exposure, and much used for building in Italy. 'It was far less crystalline than most of the Italian travertin.' He also saw quartz, schist (kinds of foliated rock containing minerals), porphyry, marble, flint, and haematite. Portions of stalactites of various sizes were strewn about near some rivers, in the beds of which were many coloured, water-smoothed and polished pebbles of various kinds. Some were of chalcedony (precious stones of the quartz type, e.g. agate).

They passed near a series of flat-topped conical hills where the ground was littered with fragments of coloured agate. The hills were of white limestone, 'much resembling chalk . . . [the tops] determined by a thick bed of silicious or cherty character'. He was reminded of the hard chalk near the Giant's Causeway in Ireland, and of 'the cones of earth left by our excavators . . .'.

With Dr Forbes, one evening, he explored some ridges and hills where various forms of quartz abounded—including some layers of 'petunse pent-landica'. On the following day, with Mr Fairley, they found fragments of 'magnetic iron ore, and we found that it sensibly affected the compass'. They also found what appeared to be 'hornblende . . . but which resembled the black augite of Stromboli . . .'. There was felspar, but no gold; 'neither with the naked eye nor with a lens did I perceive the smallest particle'. On one hill there were masses of marble, and great veins of it interspersed with carbonate of lime. There were signs that the marble had been quarried; there were cuts and grooves in the slabs, where, in all probability, wooden wedges had been driven. When watered the wood would swell and cleave the stone. One piece of marble was clearly 'designed for a column ten feet long . . .' but Hodgkin never saw examples of the use of marble, 'either in ancient or modern work' in the country.

Well, we now know that minerals of many sorts are mined in Morocco and that their 'phosphate plateau' in this area is the world's largest deposit. Exploitation began in 1921, Hodgkin would have been interested to learn. As he said, 'It is a part of the country which merits careful geological examination'.

MARRAKESH

As they crossed the plain, the snow-covered peaks of the Atlas range came into view. Marrakesh lay in a broad valley between the mountains and the 'Jiblet Hills', and the tall (230 feet) Koutoubia tower could be seen for many miles. It is all that remains of a twelfth century mosque. Around it rose other smaller minarets; great palm trees came in sight. Nearing the city, horsemen came galloping out, followed by Jews mounted on mules and asses; there were also curious Moors. They crossed a river on a fine old bridge of 'twenty spans' and 'pointed piers', to enter a pleasant place of gardens, little streams and heavily-laden date palms; 'everything nice and green'.

'Passing the city walls by a small gate we saw before us a loftier wall, with a large ornamented Moorish gateway'. This proved to be the entrance to the citadel. Turning left they came to 'a large oblong arena . . . a grand resort for horse soldiers, who spend hours there in that display of galloping and firing which, by English travellers, is called "powder play"'. This may have been the great Djemaa el Fna Square, where, today, of an evening, the story-tellers, acrobats, sword swallowers, and snake charmers gather, to entertain, not only the natives, but the visitors from Holiday Inn.

The party were conducted to 'a quadrangular house or palace' where they were to be accommodated. It was in the middle of a much neglected garden, although it was well stocked with orange and lemon trees. The house had three storeys and an inner courtyard open to the sky, but 'it had a close and musty odour', suggesting damp. It lacked tables and chairs; there were no fireplaces or glass windows. The nights were cold and they were all rather disappointed. However, there were new Brussel carpets on the floors, European bedsteads, pillows, glassware and 'a good deal of finery and effect in inferior workmanship'.

For some days they saw little of the actual city, as they were confined to their house while they waited, in the customary manner, for the Sultan to send for them. This was 'quite a trial', but Hodgkin got out on a few occasions to see patients. One was the Prime Minister, and another was one of his friends. Hodgkin said nothing about the nature of their complaints. What little he saw of the city, he did not like. It was 'dirty but large,' with thick, high walls of 'beaten earth', narrow ways, vacant spaces, markets, and mosques. Outside the city walls were 'banks of debris', carcasses and skeletons of animals, many pits, and the ruins and refuse of ages.

On 31 January they were informed that the Sultan would see them at half-past seven the following morning, so 'we had to be stirring early . . .'. The Prime Minister and the Chamberlain came to conduct them, Sir Moses in his sedan and the remainder of the company on horses or mules. They had about half a mile to go to 'the imperial premises', 'we did not go into, or even in sight of, the palace'. Their route was lined with strange-looking troops, old and young, fair and dark, many with shaven heads. Few had shoes, trousers were short and baggy, jackets were red, blue, or green. 'These troops had very much the appearance of prisoners clothed in left off soldiers' garments', but each of them had a musket.

In the courtyard, where the Sultan came riding in through an archway, on a fine, white prancing horse, the soldiers were better turned out. The interview 'was not a long one . . .'. The Emperor was about forty-five, dark but not black, and his features were not negroid; 'forehead good'. He was marked by smallpox and had an impediment of speech, 'which is slow and constantly interrupted by a noise, compared by some to a bark . . .'. He was reputed to be a mathematician.

On a second visit they were received in the Sultan's 'domain', a sort of 'Moorish Champ de Mars', beyond the arched gateway in the picture. Here again, they had to wait in a room which appeared to be 'an office for scribes'. Then they were taken to an 'extensive garden of orange, lemon, olive and other trees, till we came to a large summer-house or pavilion', where the Sultan was sitting on a raised divan. 'This was the only apartment into which we were admitted.' Its floor and walls were covered with a rich mosaic of minute glazed tiles, green predominating. They later spent several hours riding in this walled domain which seemed 'to unite the character of garden, orchard and field'. There were lakes and pools, olive groves and vineyards, and extensive irrigation. At no time did they obtain a view of 'the imperial residence' and they concluded that the domain must have been very extensive.

One afternoon, after riding through the city, a dust storm blew up, and a cold wind came in from the desert. In the distance there appeared to be 'a brownish fog', and rain fell. It took some time and care to cleanse themselves, and Hodgkin wondered what part such storms played in causing the widespread ophthalmia.

On another day, he says in his geological addendum, they were taken to 'the Imperial estate', which consisted of fields, olive and orange groves, water courses, and lakes frequented by game. They had guns and greyhounds, but Hodgkin preferred to wander off towards a 'Mahometan's Saint's Tomb, or sacred house'. He was not allowed to enter it, as his soldier-guide indicated that it was a place of reverence, forbidden to visitors.

By contrast with all the richness and space, the Jewish quarter, which Sir Moses stoutly penetrated with difficulty on his sedan, was poor and densely populated. One of the synagogues was visited and many rabbis were called on. They were entertained at the home of one of the wealthier Jews.

MARRAKESH TO JADIDA

They left Marrakesh on 8 February, travelling northwestwards, across the river Tensift and the Jiblet hills, through the cultivated province of Doukkala, to El Jadida on the Atlantic coast, about sixty-five miles south of Casablanca. For this journey they used mules only, 'giving up camels for the tents and baggage, and horses for riding'. Consul Reade, however, retained his horse. Hodgkin was thrown from his mule while he was sketching, as the result of a mule driver's clumsiness. He continued the day's journey on foot, 'which gave me the opportunity of quitting the path to examine objects on the way'. The eyes of the geologist were alert all the way to the coast. He concluded that the gritty character of Moroccan bread was due to the use of granite in making millstones. There were more conical hills with flat tops, more limestone and quartz, and at one place, buried in the travertin, he found 'crystals of dog-tooth spar'. What joy!

Place names mentioned were Boo Limoor, Sahrij, Shishowa, and

Smira. One day it was cold and rainy. Water was satisfactory except at one well, where it was thick and brownish. They rigged up a filter from a towel, pebbles, and charcoal.

In a kaid's enclosure Hodgkin found that a broth of goat meat and flour was 'by no means unpleasant'. In a citadel of the Pacha of Doukkala they were accommodated, with their tents, in a garden; they were also allotted three pavilions. Sir Moses was presented with a horse. There was no invitation to enter the actual residence of the kaid or of the pacha.

As they approached the old Portuguese port of Mazagan (El Jadida), they were met by English and European officials and merchants and 'a motley assemblage . . . of young and old, rich and poor, male and female, either going on foot, or mounted on horses, mules or donkeys, with or without saddles, and in some instances two on the same beast, whilst their costume was quite as varied . . .'. There was much noise, 'especially that produced by the vibratory motion of the tongue, as expressive of joy'.

At El Jadida, HMS *Magicienne* lay off port. They had 'a capital repast, at a well-supplied table, at which were good wines of several kinds', at the house of the Vice-Consul. It was a well constructed building, based on an old Portuguese church; the Union Jack flew from its tower. There were ramparts by the sea, ruins of old fortifications and a remarkable underground reservoir. This was of Portuguese construction, and thought to have once been an armoury. The 'citerne' is still there. With its arches and pillars, and with light entering from a circular opening in the roof, it resembles a flooded church crypt.

They steamed off to Tangier the same evening, and on arrival Hodgkin and a few of the officers went ashore with the help of the waders. Sir Moses was fatigued and remained on board. Hodgkin wished to inspect the ruins of an old Roman bridge. He walked the two miles to it, over rough ground, and returned to enjoy 'an excellent dinner' on board, while they sailed to Gibraltar. There, they spent 'several days pleasantly' with an enjoyable farewell dinner.

Although the brilliant result of an arduous mission, undertaken under circumstances of sorrow and gloom, tended in no small degree to infuse a joyful feeling as we were seated at a sumptuous repast, there was nevertheless a prevailing seriousness at the approaching separation of so many sympathising friends.

'Poor speaker that I am', Hodgkin said, of that occasion, 'I could not remain silent . . .'.

THE JOURNEY HOME

They embarked on a French steam packet for Malaga on 25 February and, travelling on to Granada by road, arrived there on the twenty-seventh. They visited the Alhambra, 'of which the specimen in the Crystal Palace gives a favourable and pretty accurate idea, except that it is on a reduced scale'. In Granada, Mr Samuel had 'a return of an old and very painful malady [which] made travelling, and even sight-seeing, distressing'. (They say in Morocco that their saddles can actually cure an attack of piles.)

They continued by road, across the Sierra Morena, to the railhead at Santa Cruz de Mudela. Sir Moses could not spend more than six hours a day in their carriage and suitable accommodation was difficult to find. 'Spanish inns, without fireplaces and with poor windows and doors, and brick floors, are not productive of creaturely comfort.' The train took them to Madrid, where Sir Moses had a second audience with the Queen on 18 March, presenting her with a copy of the edict he had obtained from the Sultan of Morocco. He had informed the latter that he had obtained assurances concerning the rights of Jews, from the Sultan of Turkey. The edict he obtained in Marrakesh stated that

. . . in the administration of the Courts of Law, the Jews shall occupy a position of perfect equality with all other people, so that not even a fractional portion of the smallest imaginable particle of injustice shall reach any of them, nor shall they be subjected to anything of an objectionable nature.

While they were in Madrid, Hodgkin chose to visit the waterworks, which were managed by a young friend from Cornwall. With him, and Mr Samuel, he spent a day in Toledo. 'It stands on an elevated situation at the extremity of a range of hills, from which it is cut off by a chasm, through which the Tagus flows, having a hill with a fortress on its summit on the left, and the city with its ruined palace on the right.' They met a clergyman from Manchester 'who was spending the winter in the south on account of his health'. In the cathedral they climbed up to the bell tower and had a fine view of the surrounding countryside. One of the bells had been cracked, and 'to counteract the effects of this, and aperture had been cut, about an inch in breadth, through about half the height of the bell'. The clappers, and not the bells, were swung.

Examining the many side-chapels and tombs, Hodgkin noticed that one tomb, 'of a fighting bishop', had 'a crescent of his coat of arms'. He commented that in the cathedral at Sienna he had seen 'a similar crescent on the escutcheon of Pope Aeneas Sylvius, a Siennese'. There was also in the cathedral at Toledo 'a very remarkable piece of Roman

Catholic superstition'. It consisted of a representation of the Virgin, with a stone 'worn by the touches of the deluded'. There was also 'a representation of a child crucified, his side cut open, his heart removed and held in the hand of the executioner—and artistic effort of deceiving and deceived priests to incense their followers against the persecuted Jews'.

They admired the Moorish tiles in an adjacent square tower and examined specimens and fragments of early art in a museum. 'Some had the delicacy and minute execution of miniatures.' In a painting of Saint George and the dragon, the former had a pair of scales in one hand, and a sword in the other; the dragon was about the size of a small dog. Of this strange painting, Hodgkin wrote

It struck me that perhaps Milton might have seen a grotesque painting of this kind and from it, might have taken the grand idea of the exhibition of Satan's impending fall in Libra, as he was about contending with the angel in Paradise, on being detected suggesting crime, in a dream, at the ear of Eve.

One is left wondering what his Victorian readers made of that thought.

They wandered along the terrace outside the town walls, inspected some Roman stonework—arched passages and terraces which suggested a former circus or amphitheatre—and looked at the old churches and synagogues. Hodgkin tested some examples of the celebrated Toledo Swords, 'of such a temper that they may be bent double . . . or struck through a silver coin without breaking'.

But sightseeing was now over. They left Madrid by the train on 20 March and were in Paris late on the 24th, travelling by diligence, as before, part of the way through Bayonne to Bordeaux. On 1 April, 'a little after one-o-clock', Hodgkin accompanied Sir Moses to the Tuileries for an audience with the French Emperor. They had to wait as 'the Emperor had been a little delayed at his breakfast'. However, he received them 'most graciously' and accepted a copy of the firman from the Sultan of Morocco.

After this successful termination of the mission we left Paris and soon arrived safely home.

Among the addenda at the end of the book there is a copy of the letter which Sir Moses sent to the Jewish community of Morocco, on his return; and a copy of a short address Hodgkin gave in Tangier; some travel notes by Mr Fairley in north Morocco; and some from a Captain Hood, from the Embassy staff in Tangier. The travel notes have a livelier tone than Hodgkin's.

Fairley visited Alcazar (Ksar El Kebir), Mequinez (Meknes) and Fez. Forty miles south of Tangier he saw the prehistoric stones 'of a Druidical character', now usually referred to as the *Stone Circle of M'Zora*. They bear some resemblance to Stonehenge. Moulay Idriss, 'romantically situated on the side of a mountain', surrounded by olive groves and with plentiful water, he was not allowed to enter. It was forbidden to Christians and Jews. It takes its name from the founder of Fez and of Morocco's first ruling dynasty. The town may now be visited and for the past twenty years, photography has been permitted. Fairley found Fez the most business-like of Morocco's cities; the streets were wider and cleaner, one a 'facsimile of that in Cordoba'. Everywhere, were gardens and fruit groves.

At a banquet in Marrakesh, Fairley enjoyed 'kabobs' (kebabs) and 'koosko-soo' (couscous). The former consisted of the now well-known spiced meats on skewers, roasted over charcoal embers. 'These things are particularly nice', he said, 'and were some enterprising cook-shop keeper to introduce them to London, I think a fortune would be the result'. He liked the couscous but found the manner of eating it a bit difficult. Dipping his hand in the dish, rolling the mass into a ball, and trying to toss it into his mouth, he usually only succeeded in getting it on to his beard, and he had to call for a spoon, amid much laughter. The dish was made from 'coarsely-ground wheat and not unlike sago before it is boiled'. Like 'the porridge of Scotland', couscous was the 'national dish'.

Captain Hood's contribution was based on a journey he made with the British ambassador from Tangier to Meknes, in 1861. It was an official visit to the Sultan and took a month; Hodgkin said that Hood was the photographer of the party. He had plenty to record; hundreds of wild mounted tribesmen, 'fine and handsome'; village bazaars, 'minarets rising from amidst the masses of white houses and red walls'; and rivers and hills to cross. At Meknes, Moorish etiquette required them to wait in their quarters for several days, as had Hodgkin and Montefiore, before the Sultan recieved them. From the top of their house they had hoped to get a view of the town 'and of the Moorish beauties', but the high parapet and narrow loop-holes, hindered them. But, he said, 'with our glasses we are enabled to discover some nice-looking women'.

At the Sultan's ceremony, before breakfast, the soldiers paraded in 'green knickerbockers, blue and red coats and Fez caps . . .'. Behind the mounted Sultan was the state executioner with his sword, followed by an official carrying 'the Sheriffian umbrella'. 'The Sultan', he wrote, 'is the only follower of the prophet who is allowed to shelter himself from the rays of the sun with an umbrella'. They subsequently visited the gardens and were presented with four ostrich eggs 'which formed a gigantic omelette, in taste like that of other eggs'. They were not allowed to visit Fez, thirty miles away, 'reputedly the finest town in the north', as 'the governor being dead the people were unruly'. They were entertained in various ways. Snake charmers were brought one day, 'thirty dirty men with a basket of snakes and two large tambourines'. 'I bought some "keef" which has the same effect on the Moors as opium has on the Chinese. It had no effect on me.'

The Sultan also sent along some members of a religious sect—the 'Hamacha'—to amuse them. They watched from the gallery, with their soldiers on guard on the steps. The leader was a negro 'in an old leathern tunic and a leopard skin, his cap embroidered in coweries and ostrich feathers'. He began responding to the drumming and eventually became 'perfectly rabid'. He was howling and shouting and dancing, slashing his head with a sword. Ultimately, one of the visiting party's servants joined in. He threw off his clothes, danced wildly, but 'his principal fancy was to get earthen pots, throw them high in the air, and let them fall on his head'. When a pot was too heavy to lift, he 'went at it like a ram, and sent his head through it. He cut himself badly at this game'. The negro also held a flame under his chin and behind his knees. The group finished up 'by wallowing in the fountain'. Hood was given to understand that all those involved were Mahommedans, but that the ceremony had nothing to do with Islamism. He was also told that no other Christian had seen it.

On putting down this book of Hodgkin's one's first thought is that it probably proved of most interest to those who wished to know about the mission to Marrakesh, than to the general reader, curious about the country of Morocco. Hodgkin's devotion to Montefiore comes through quite clearly. Theirs was one of those rare friendships which link men of different temperaments. Yet, from the book itself, one learns little about them. One would like also to have an account of the journey by some other member of the party—someone who might have told us more about these two so dissimilar persons—the tycoon and the puritan. We can judge that Montefiore was a powerful personality, full of good will and determination, and that Hodgkin was energetic and, in his own way, very observant. But he sounds a dry old stick and his prose is not attractive.

The reader may well get a picture of the landscape of that part of Morocco, with its advancing wind-blown sands, the buried palaces and the forlorn rubbishy ruins, but there is very little about the people and their mode of life. One wonders if he ever tried a kebab or couscous. And as for Catholic Spain, it clearly made him shudder. We can see him frowning at a baroque facade or wrinkling his nose at candles or incense.

But there is no denying the significance of his geological observations. They constitute the most original feature of the book. Although he had journeyed widely in many countries, over many years, he had not published any other book of travel. When he came to write about the road to Marrakesh, we see that he lacked those gifts of humour and imagination so desirable in the travel writer—and so often witheld from the Messrs. Valiant for Truth of this world.

The writer first learned of Dr Thomas Hodgkin, the traveller, in Jaffa, Palestine, in 1942, when he was stationed at a British military hospital in nearby Sarafand. One of the Jewish Palestinian doctors at the hospital took me to Hodgkin's grave in the little English cemetery after we had been swimming at the officers' beach club in Jaffa. There was a granite obelisk, suitably inscribed, giving the date of his death as the fourth of April 1866. It also recorded that the monument had been erected by Sir Moses Montefiore Bart., 'in commemmoration of a friendship of more than forty years, and of many journeys taken together in Europe, Asia and Africa'.

BIBLIOGRAPHY

British Medical Journal. Obituary of Dr. T. Hodgkin. *Br. Med. J.* i, 447 (1866).
Dictionary of National Biography. Dr. T. Hodgkin. Vol. 27, p. 63 (1891).
Foxon, G.E.H. Thomas Hodgkin, 1798–1866; a biographical note. *Guy's Hosp. Rep.* **115**, 243 (1966).
Hancock, P. E. T. Thomas Hodgkin. *J. R. Coll. Physns. Lond.* **2**, 404 (1968).
Rose, Michael. *Curator of the dead: Thomas Hodgkin (1798–1866).* Peter Owen, London (1981).
Rosenbloom, J. An interesting friendship—Thomas Hodgkin MD and Sir Moses Montefiore, Bart. *Ann. Med. Hist.* **3**, 381 (1921).
Sakula, A. Dr. Thomas Hodgkin and Sir Moses Montefiore Bart—the friendship of two remarkable men. *J. R. Soc. Med.* **72**, 382 (1979).
Stern, E.S. Dr. Hodgkin's relationship with his distinguished friend and patient, Sir Moses Montefiore, Bt., FRS. *Med. Hist.* **II**, 182 (1967).

Index